Original first edition

ISBN: 978-3-98929-291-8

Imprint:
Book Shelter GmbH
Aufhäuserstrasse 64
30457 Hanover
Germany

Yoga and Christmas: A Harmonious Blend

The holiday season is a time of joy, connection, and generosity, but it can also be one of the busiest, most stressful times of the year. Between gift shopping, family gatherings, travel, and the natural shift of seasons, many people find themselves overwhelmed, stretched thin, and running on autopilot.

Yoga offers us an antidote to this. Just as Christmas reminds us of light, hope, and togetherness, yoga grounds us in presence, balance, and renewal. Both traditions call us to slow down, look inward, and reconnect to what truly matters. By weaving yoga into the holiday season, we create a sanctuary for ourselves; a reminder that peace is found not in what we do, but in how we choose to be.

This Yoga Advent Calendar is designed to bring these worlds together: the sacred pause of yoga, and the festive spirit of the holidays. Each day becomes not just a countdown to Christmas, but a journey inward, a daily gift of presence, peace, and grounding.

Why This Practice Matters During the Holidays

December often feels like a blur. The to-do lists are long, the calendar is full, and expectations, both from ourselves and others, can weigh heavily on us. While we may love the lights, music, and traditions, it's easy to get lost in the rush.

That's where this advent calendar comes in. It offers a reminder that even five minutes of stillness, breath, or mindful movement can completely shift your day. These practices are not about perfection or complexity; they're about anchoring yourself amidst the whirlwind.

Imagine pausing each morning or evening, unrolling your mat, and giving yourself the gift of a short, simple yoga practice. In that moment, the noise fades, and you return to your body, your breath, and your heart. That's what this calendar is about: a chance to slow down, breathe, and remember the deeper joy of the season.

What You'll Find Inside

Each day of the Advent calendar brings you something new; something simple, accessible, and grounding. You don't need any prior yoga experience to follow along. The practices are designed for beginners, though seasoned practitioners will also find comfort and joy in their simplicity.

- **Gentle Yoga Flows:** Short sequences to release tension and move your body with ease.
- **Breathwork Practices:** Simple breathing techniques to calm the mind and settle holiday stress.
- **Meditations:** Guided moments of stillness to bring you back to presence and gratitude.
- **Yin-Style Holds:** Longer, supported poses to release deep layers of tension and invite relaxation.

Each practice takes **five minutes or less**, making it realistic to fit into even the busiest of days. This isn't another task on your list; it's a tool to help you maneuver through the holidays with more calm, clarity, and joy.

The Gift of Presence

Yoga teaches us that the most precious gift we can offer is presence—presence with ourselves, and presence with others. This advent calendar isn't just about stretching or breathing. It's about creating a small ritual of self-care that allows you to show up more fully for the people and moments that matter most.

When you take five minutes to ground yourself, you carry that calm into the rest of your day. Conversations feel lighter, holiday errands feel less stressful, and even the quiet moments like watching snow fall outside your window or sipping a warm drink become more vivid, joyful, and meaningful.

This season, instead of being swept away by the chaos, you get to root yourself in peace. This is the true gift of yoga during the Christmas season: learning how to stay centered, grounded, and open-hearted amidst it all.

About Me

I have been practicing yoga for over 15 years; and teaching for 10. My journey has taken me across **Canada, the USA, and India**, where I've trained in multiple traditions and styles, accumulating over **500 hours of formal yoga training**.

Yoga has been my anchor, my teacher, and my greatest source of balance. While I love sharing the practice with others, I also keep a strong personal self-practice that nourishes me daily. This foundation allows me to show up for my students with authenticity, groundedness, and clarity.

I teach both **online and in-person practices**, and my teaching style blends tradition with accessibility. My intention is always to make yoga feel welcoming, approachable, and supportive for every student, whether it's their first class or their thousandth.

This advent calendar is a reflection of my heart and my teaching: yoga that is simple, grounding, and deeply supportive of your everyday life. I hop that these practices bring you moments of peace, presence, and joy throughout this holiday season.

Week 1:
AWAKEN

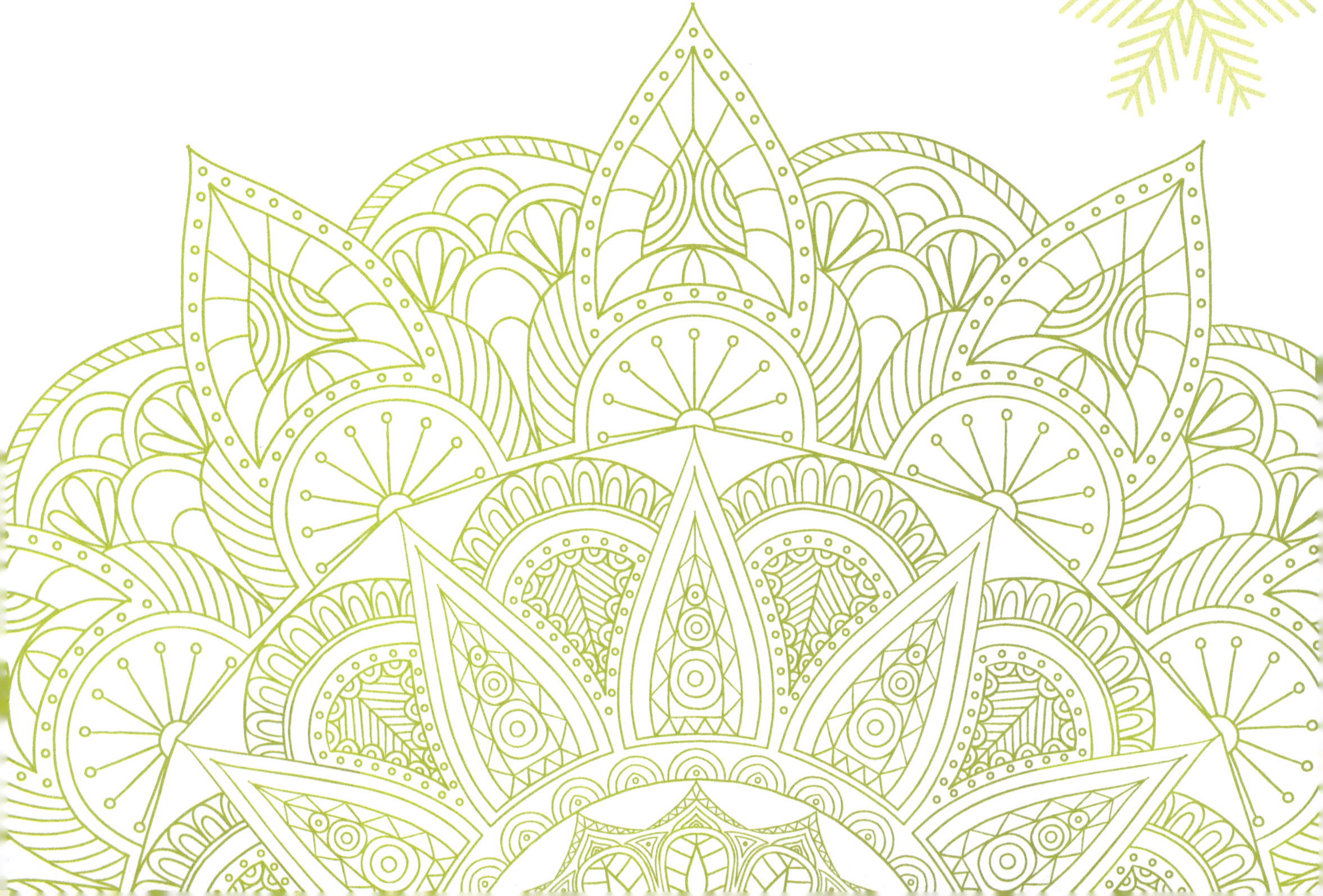

Quote of the Week:

"The soul awakens; when the mind softens."

The journey of your Yoga Advent Calendar begins with awakening. But awakening here doesn't mean pushing, striving, or forcing yourself into action. Instead, it is a gentle call to open, like the slow unfurling of a flower or the quiet rising of the sun. Awakening is about becoming more present, more aware, and more connected to yourself, even in the midst of this season's busyness.

During the holidays, our minds can become full, with lists to check off, people to see, and endless tasks to complete. When the mind is cluttered, it's easy to lose touch with the soul. This week's theme reminds us that true awakening doesn't come from adding more to our plates, but from softening, slowing down, and allowing space for our inner wisdom to surface. As the quote says, *"The soul awakens, when the mind softens."* By letting go of tension, distraction, and mental noise, we make room for clarity, calm, and connection.

In these first six days, you'll be guided through simple practices (gentle yoga flows, calming breathwork, meditations, and yin-inspired holds) that invite you to reawaken your body and your spirit. Each one takes less than five minutes, making them accessible no matter how busy your days feel. Think of them as small daily rituals: a pause to awaken your breath, awareness, and heart.

This week is about noticing subtle shifts. As you step onto your mat each day, you may begin to feel lighter in your body, steadier in your mind, and more grounded in your heart. Awakening is not about a grand transformation all at once; it's about small moments of awareness that build over time. Even a few minutes of presence can change the energy of your entire day.

As you move through days 1–6, approach each practice with curiosity and softness. Let your breath guide you. Let your body move with ease, and let your mind quiet just enough to hear the whispers of your soul. This is where the awakening begins.

Day 1

Theme of the Week: Awaken
Quote of the Week: "The soul awakens when the mind softens."

Theme of the Day: Begin Within
Quote of the Day: "You are the light you seek."

Yoga for Spinal Wake-Up

Our journey begins not with outward movement, but with an inward turning. Before we step into the world, we start by listening; feeling the body's rhythms, noticing the breath, and honoring the space between each inhale and exhale. Today's gentle sequence will awaken your spine, melt away morning stiffness, and ground you in quiet presence, setting a steady tone for the day ahead.

Cat–Cow Flow

Come to a tabletop position, hands planted beneath shoulders, knees beneath hips. Spread your fingers wide and feel your palms root into the earth. Take a moment to close your eyes; and feel the natural rhythm of your breath.

On an inhale, move into *Cow Pose*: soften your belly toward the mat, lift your chest and gaze, and gently draw your heart forward. Feel the front of your body expand.

Exhale into *Cat Pose*: press the ground away, round your spine toward the ceiling, and tuck your chin to your chest. Let your shoulder blades spread, releasing any tension.

Flow slowly between these shapes for 5 mindful rounds, letting your breath guide the movement.

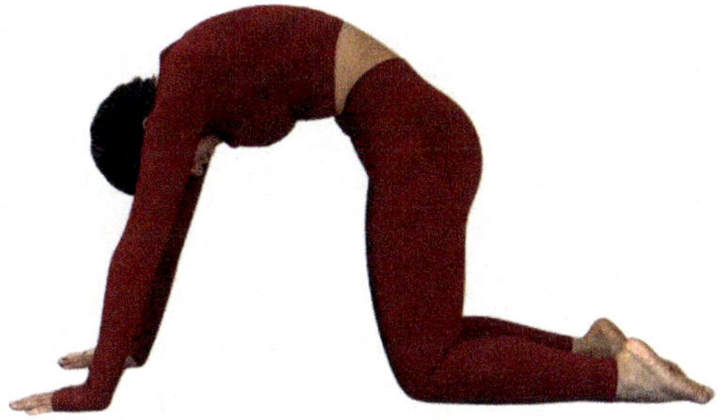

Cat Pose

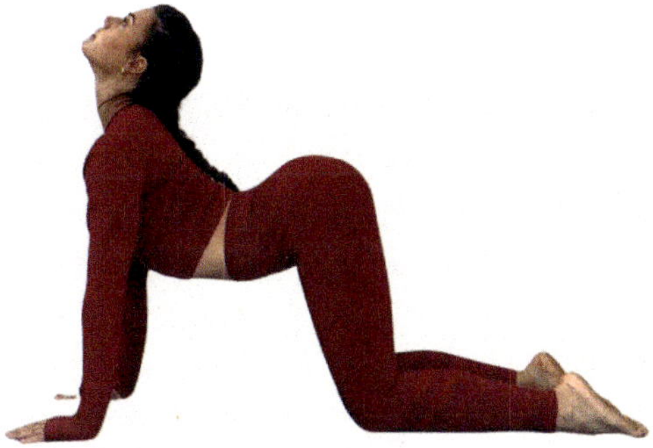

Cow Pose

Child's Pose

After your final round, ease back into *Child's Pose*. Spread knees wide, touch your big toes together, and walk your the fingertips forward as you sit your hips to your heels. Ground your forehead to the mat, allowing your body to surrender into the earth. Take 10 deep breaths, feeling the back expand on the inhale and soften on the exhale.

Here, in this stillness, remember: every journey begins within—and you already carry the light you seek.

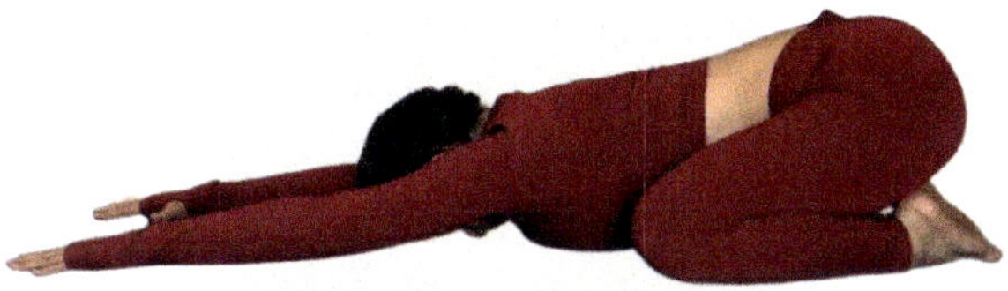

Child's Pose

Day 2

Theme of the Week: Awaken
Quote of the Week: "The soul awakens when the mind softens."

Theme of the Day: Rise with Ease
Quote of the Day: "Start where you are, soften into the moment, and let the day unfold."

Seated Morning Stretch

This morning, we greet the day with gentleness. Rather than rushing forward, we create space—space in the body for breath to flow freely, and space in the mind for clarity to emerge. Today's practice will awaken your spine, lengthen your side body, and release tension in the neck, leaving you grounded, refreshed, and ready to meet the day with lightness.

Sit in a comfortable cross-legged position, on a mat or cushion. Let your hands rest on your knees, close your eyes, and notice your breath as it is—no need to change it yet.

Seated Cat–Cow

Inhale, draw your heart forward, and roll your shoulders back, letting your chest open fully.

Exhale, round through your spine, tuck your chin toward your chest, and gently engage your core.

Flow slowly between these shapes for 5 rounds, letting your breath lead the movement.

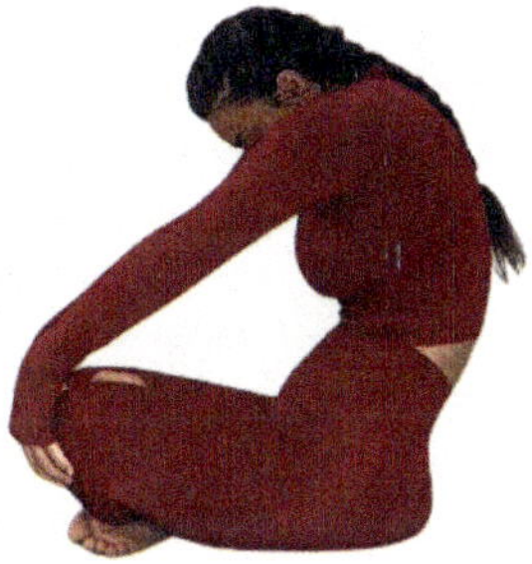

Seated Cat

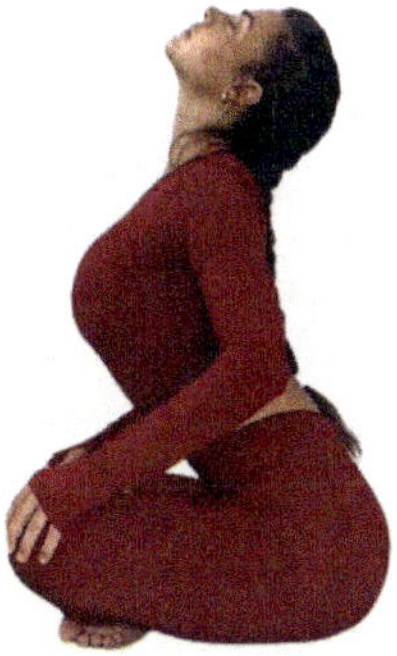

Seated Cow

Side Bends

Place your right hand on the mat beside you. Inhale, lift your left arm toward the sky, lengthening through the ribs.

Exhale, lean to the right, and feel the stretch along your left side. Brea-the here for 5 steady breaths. Switch sides.

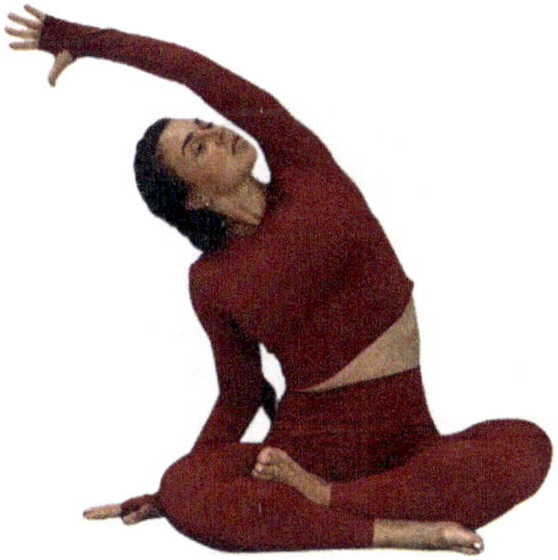

Side Bends

Neck Stretch

Drop your right ear toward your right shoulder. Bring your right arm up and over your head and rest your right hand lightly over your left ear for a gentle deepening-do not force it, use only gentle pressure. Hold for 5 slow breaths, softening the neck and shoulders. Switch sides.

As you rise from your seat, carry this sense of ease forward, letting your day unfold in its own perfect rhythm.

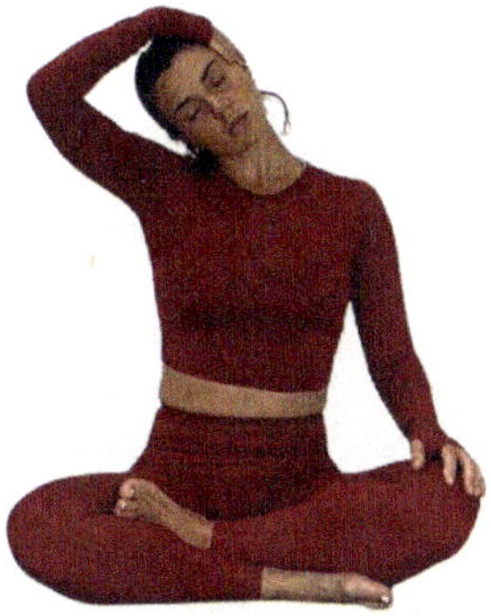

Neck Stretch

Day 3

Theme of the Week: Awaken
Quote of the Week: "The soul awakens when the mind softens."

Theme of the Day: Move Like Water
Quote of the Day: "Flow, don't force."

Standing Flow

Today we invite movement to feel effortless, like water carving its path with patience and grace. Each inhale lifts and expands you, and each exhale softens and releases you. This gentle standing sequence will awaken your body, ground your energy, and draw you fully into the present moment.

Mountain Pose

Stand tall with feet hip-width apart, arms relaxed at your sides, palms open. Root down through all four corners of your feet and gently engage your legs. Lift through the crown of your head while softening your shoulders away from your ears. Take several slow breaths here, feeling steady and present.

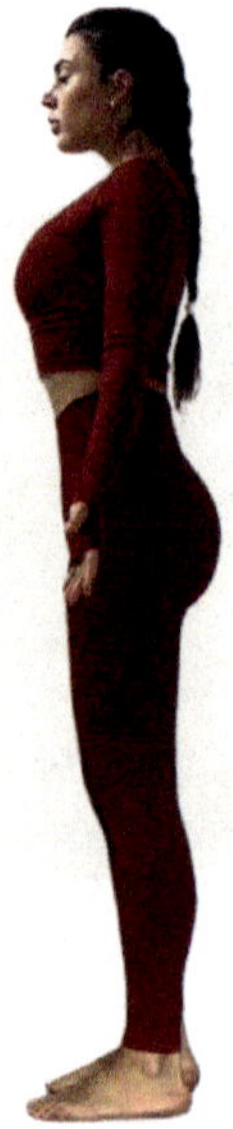

Mountain

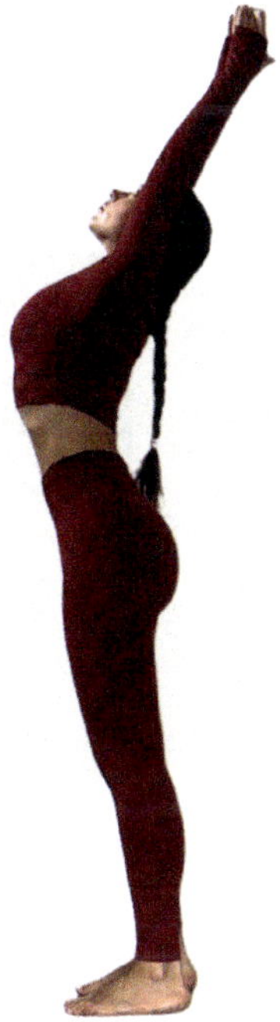

Upward Salute

Upward Salute

Inhale, sweeping your arms out and up toward the sky. Lift your gaze to meet your fingertips, lengthening through the body. Let your chest open and your ribs expand, filling your lungs.

Forward Fold

Exhale, hinging at the hips to fold over your legs. Keep a generous bend in your knees to ease the lower back. Let your head and arms hang heavy, releasing tension.

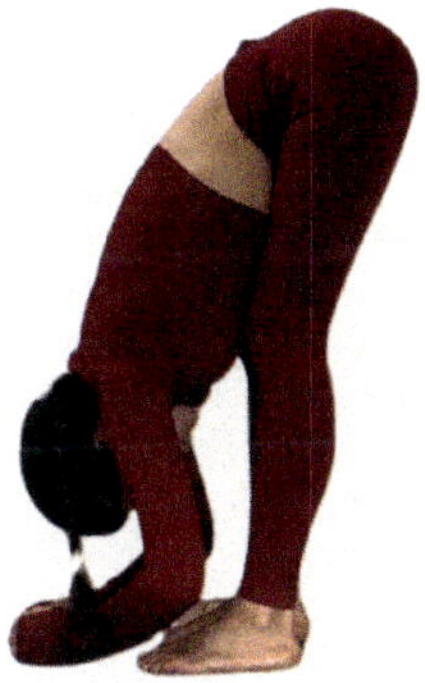

Forward Fold

Flow with Breath

From the fold, inhale and slowly roll up to standing, stacking your spine one vertebra at a time. As you rise, sweep your arms back into *Upward Salute*.

Exhale, folding forward once again.

Repeat this cycle for 5 slow, intentional rounds, letting your breath lead the way. Move like water, without strain, without rush.

When finished, return to *Mountain Pose*. Close your eyes, breathe deeply, and feel the quiet energy you've cultivated ready to ripple through the rest of your day.

Day 4

Theme of the Week: Awaken
Quote of the Week: "The soul awakens when the mind softens."

Theme of the Day: Breathe to Awaken
Quote of the Day: "Awaken the breath, and the body will follow."

Box Breathing

Today we focus on one of the most transformative yet often overlooked tools we carry everywhere: our breath. Usually, we move through the day on autopilot, taking shallow breaths that leave our body and mind undernourished. By slowing down and breathing with intention, we can shift our energy, quiet the mind, and reawaken the body's natural vitality.

Box breathing is a simple, yet powerful technique that calms the nervous system and invites balance. Imagine each inhale as a fresh wave of uplifting energy, and each exhale as a gentle release, letting go of tension, heaviness, or thoughts you no longer need.

The Breathwork Practice

Find a comfortable seat—on the floor, on a cushion, or in a chair with both feet grounded. Sit tall, lengthening your spine, and soften your shoulders away from your ears.

Close your eyes or keep a soft gaze toward the floor. Begin by exhaling fully through the nose.

- **Inhale** through your nose for a slow count of 4, letting your belly and ribs expand.
- **Hold** gently for a count of 4, resting in the stillness.
- **Exhale** through the nose for a count of 4, feeling the body soften.
- **Hold** again for a count of 4 before beginning the next breath.

Continue for 8 steady rounds. If the mind wanders, return to the rhythm of counting and the sensation of breath moving through you.

When you're finished, take a deep cleansing breath-in through the nose- out through the mouth. Then return to your natural rhythm of breathing; and notice any shifts: a calmer mind, a lighter body, or a brighter mood. Let this awakened breath carry you through the rest of your day.

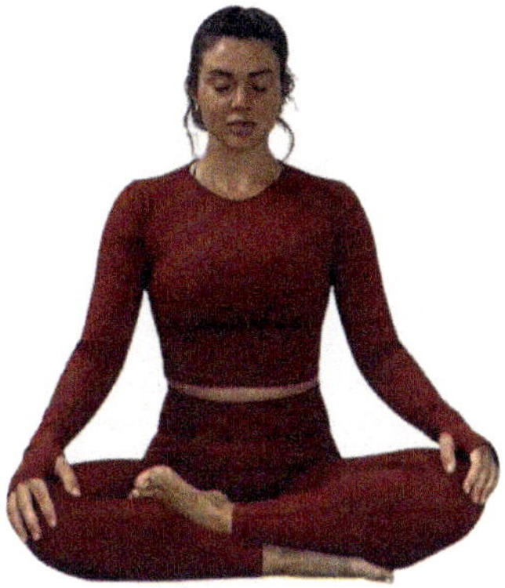

Comfortable Seat Hand to Knees

Day 5

Theme of the Week: Awaken
Quote of the Week: "The soul awakens when the mind softens."

Theme of the Day: Balance
Quote of the Day: "Balance is found in the pause."

Balancing Flow

Balance is more than holding still; it is the art of returning to center, again and again. True steadiness is found in the quiet spaces between movement, where patience and presence meet. Today's short sequence strengthens the legs and core, sharpens focus, and cultivates a grounded calm from within.

Mountain Pose

Stand tall with feet hip-width apart, arms relaxed by your sides, palms facing forward. Press evenly through both feet, lift gently through the crown of your head, and soften your shoulders away from your ears. Take several slow breaths, and anchor yourself in the present.

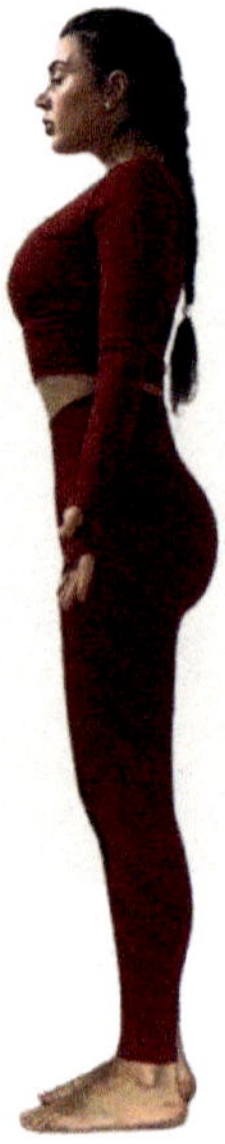

Mountain

Standing Knee to Chest-Warrior 3: Right Side Flow

Draw hands together in prayer above your heart. Inhale, shifting your weight into your left foot, *Standing Knee to Chest Pose*. Lift your right knee to hip height, spine tall.

Exhale, hinging from the hips to extend your right leg behind you into *Warrior III*. Keep your hips level and gaze down for stability.

Inhale slowly to balance as you return upright, with the right knee lifted.

Exhale, flowing back into *Warrior III*.

Repeat for 5 rounds, moving with your breath. Return to *Mountain Pose* before switching to the second side.

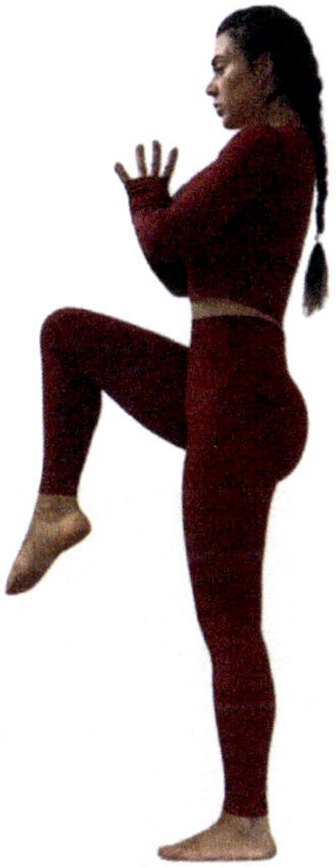

Standing Knee to Chest

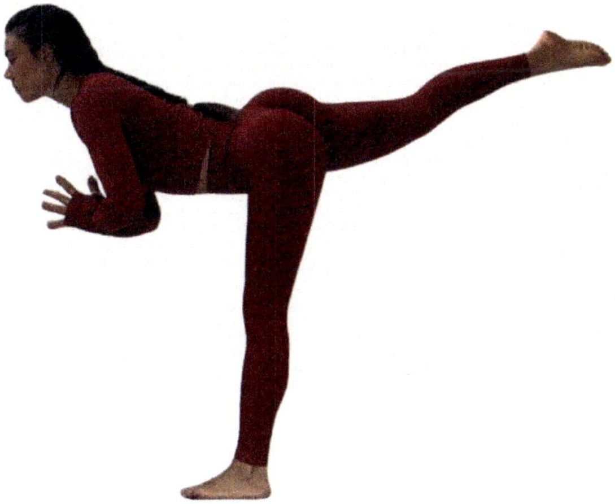

Warrior 3

Left Side Flow

Shift your weight into your right foot and mirror the sequence on the left for 5 rounds. Notice any differences in balance, strength, or focus between sides.

Return to *Mountain Pose*, standing tall and still for several breaths. Let this pause remind you: balance is not a perfect stillness; it is the practice of returning to center, no matter how many times you sway.

Day 6

Theme of the Week: Awaken
Quote of the Week: "The soul awakens when the mind softens."

Theme of the Day: Move with intention, live with purpose.
Quote of the Day: "Inhale peace, exhale tension."

Morning Intention Meditation

Before the day gathers speed, we pause, turning inward to plant the seed of intention. A few quiet minutes can shift our energy, bring clarity to the mind, and soothe the body's natural stress response. By pairing slow, mindful breathing with a clear intention, we step into the day with focus, openness, and ease.

Find a comfortable seat—on a cushion, block, or in a chair with both feet grounded. Lengthen your spine, rest your hands on your thighs or lap, and soften your shoulders. Close your eyes.

Breath Awareness

Inhale deeply through the nose, filling your lungs fully.

Exhale slowly through your nose or mouth, letting any tension melt away.

Repeat for 3 more cycles, let each inhale invite peace, and each exhale release what no longer serves you.

Set Your Intention

Let your breath settle into a natural rhythm, in and out through the nose. Ask yourself softly: *How do I want to move through this day?*

The answer may be a single word—such as *calm*, *focused*, or *kind*—or a short phrase, like *I meet the day with an open heart*. Trust whatever arises without judgment.

Silently repeat your intention with each breath. On the inhale, imagine drawing it in; on the exhale, picture it flowing through your body and out into the world.

After 2–3 minutes, take one final deep inhale, hold gently, and exhale fully. When you're ready, open your eyes, carrying your intention forward as a quiet compass to guide the day ahead.

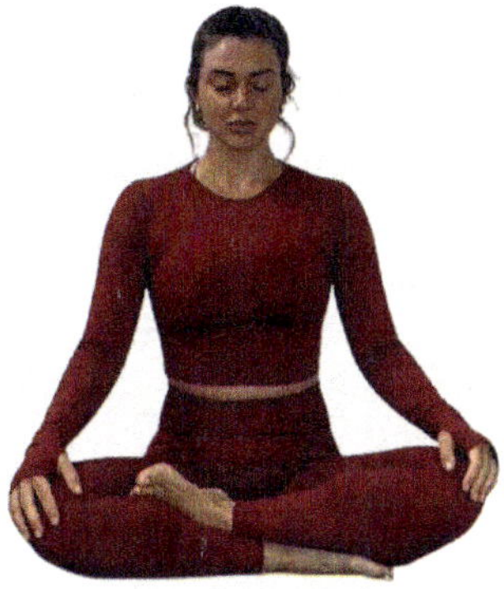

Comfortable Seat Hand to Knees

Week 2:

GROUND

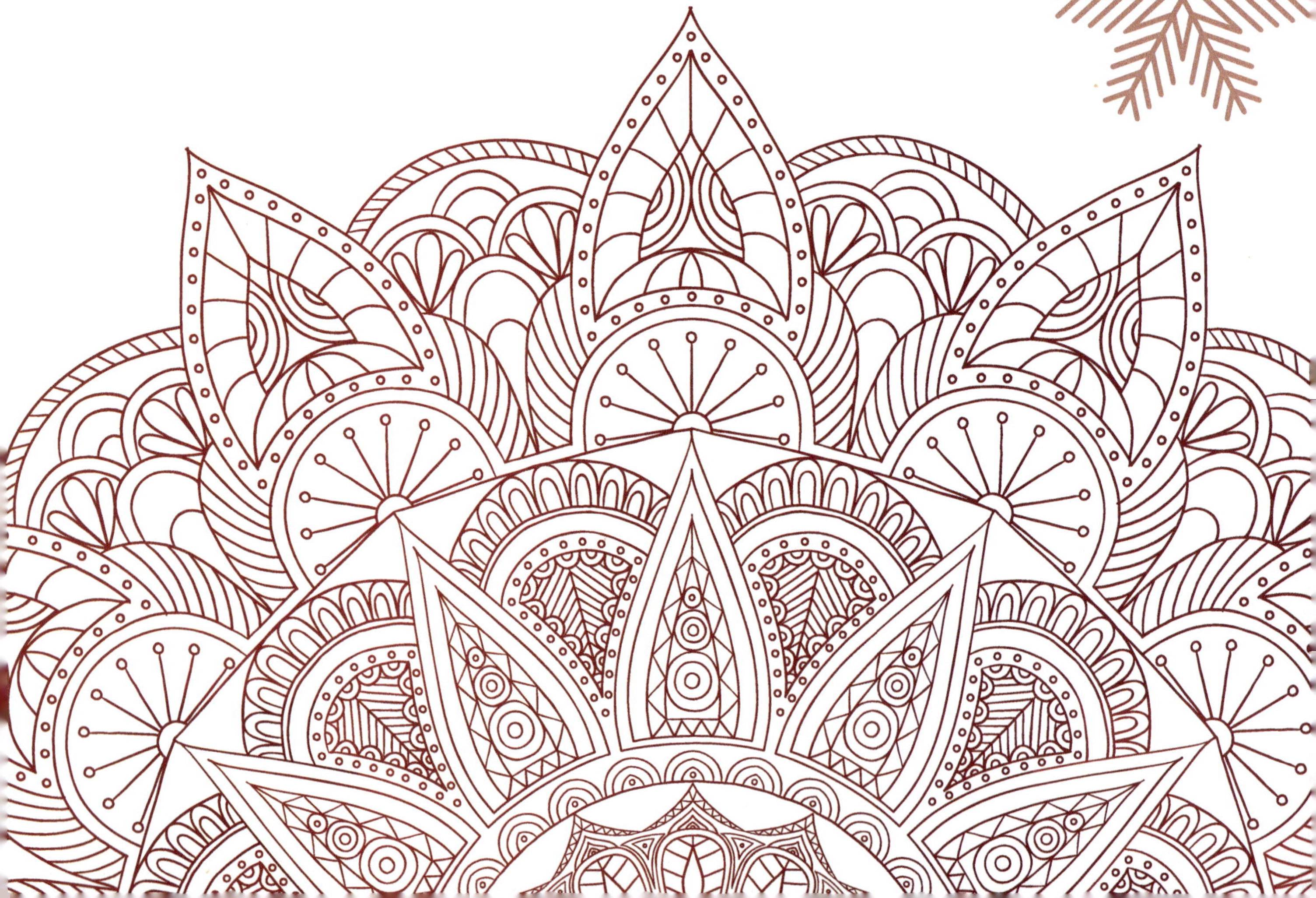

Quote of the Week:

"Root deeply, rise freely."

As we move into Week 2, the focus shifts to **grounding**. The first week awakened your awareness; now it's time to anchor it. The holiday season often pulls us in many directions: gatherings, errands, emotions, and endless to-dos. Without a steady foundation, it's easy to feel scattered and unbalanced. This week reminds us that just as a tree cannot grow tall without strong roots, we too must root ourselves deeply in presence to rise freely into the fullness of our lives.

Grounding is not only about stillness; it's about stability. When you feel grounded, your nervous system calms, your thoughts settle, and you find clarity amidst chaos. Grounding practices reconnect you with the earth beneath you, the breath within you, and the quiet strength that is always available at your core.

The practices this week will invite you to slow down, settle, and draw your energy inward. Through gentle holds, mindful breathwork, and simple postures that emphasize connection to the ground, you'll create a steady base for the rest of the season. Each short practice, whether it's a yin-style pose, a calming breath, or a meditation on stillness, becomes an anchor you can return to whenever you feel swept away.

As you move through days 7–13, notice how rooting down creates a sense of expansion. Just as the roots of a tree dig deep to nourish its growth upward, the more you connect to your foundation, the more freedom you feel to move, breathe, and live with ease. This week is your reminder that stability and freedom are not opposites; they are partners. Root deeply, and you rise naturally.

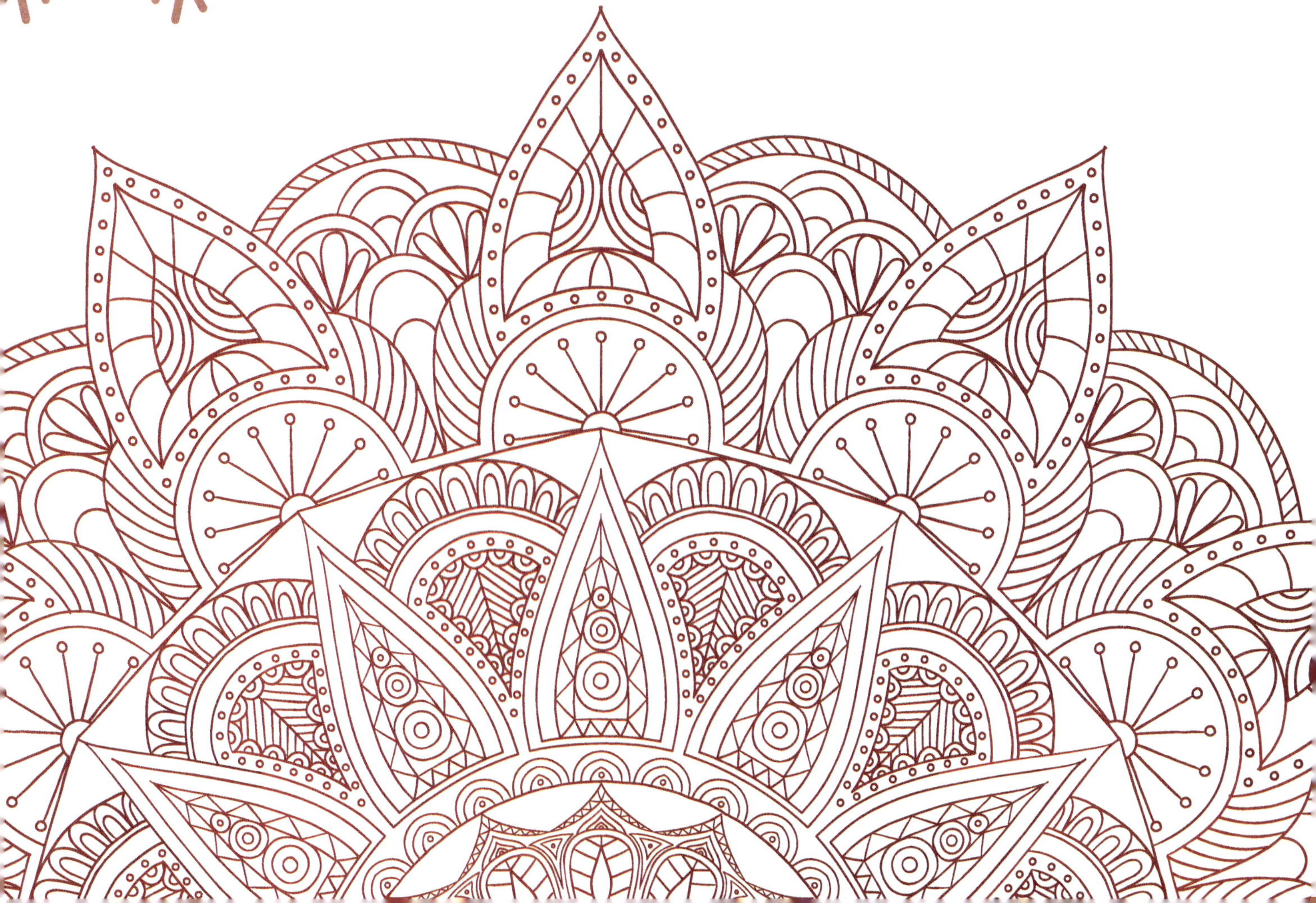

Day 7

Theme of the Week: Ground
Quote of the Week: "Root deeply, rise freely."

Theme of the Day: Strength in Stillness
Quote of the Day: "Grounded feet, open heart."

Rooted Warrior Flow

When life feels busy or uncertain, grounding ourselves through mindful movement helps us return to center. Today's practice builds both stability and openness; anchoring your body with strong, rooted legs while expanding the heart and chest with each breath. The warrior postures remind us that steadiness and openness are partners, working together to help us stand tall, present, and unshakable.

Right Side Flow

Begin in *Mountain Pose* at the top of your mat, feet grounded, spine tall, shoulders relaxed. Take two deep breaths, feeling the earth's steady support beneath you.

Step your left foot back into *Warrior II*. Align your front heel with your back arch, front knee stacked over your ankle. Press evenly into both feet, extending your arms wide, palms down. Gaze softly over your front fingertips.

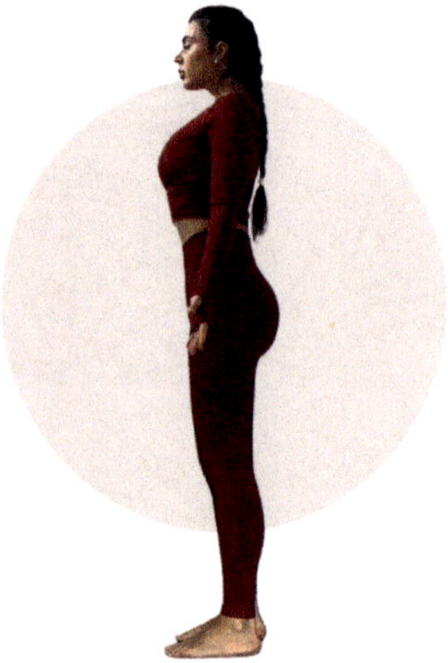

Mountain

Inhale to *Reverse Warrior*, put your left hand on your thigh as right arm reaches up and back, lengthening through the side body.

Exhale into *Extended Side Angle*, right forearm resting lightly on your thigh or hand planting to the inside of the foot, left arm extending alongside the ear.

Flow between *Reverse Warrior* on the inhale and *Extended Side Angle* on the exhale for 5 mindful rounds, feeling the strength in your legs and the openness along the side of your body.

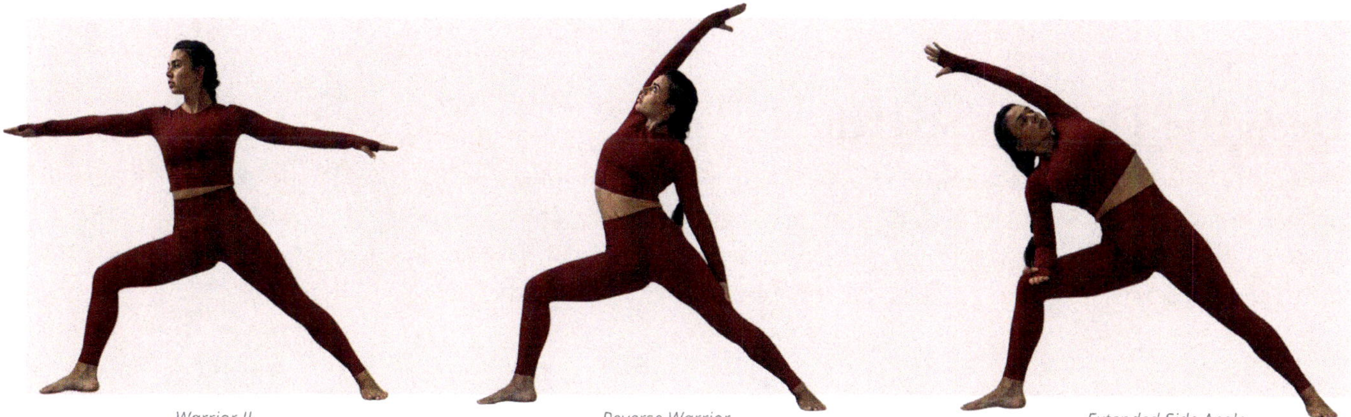

Warrior II *Reverse Warrior* *Extended Side Angle*

Left Side Flow

Return to *Mountain Pose* briefly, then step your right foot back into *Warrior II*. Repeat the same breath-led sequence for 5 rounds.

Closing

Step forward into *Mountain Pose*. Close your eyes, noticing both the grounded strength beneath you and the spaciousness within your heart. Carry this balance off the mat, rooted in your foundation, yet open to all that unfolds.

Day 8

Theme of the Week: Ground
Quote of the Week: "Root deeply, rise freely."

Theme of the Day: Grounded in Your Wholeness
Quote of the Day: "You are already enough."

Deep Hip-Opening Stretch

We often come to the mat thinking we must "fix" or "improve" something about ourselves. But yoga reminds us: you are already whole. Your breath, your body, and your presence are enough exactly as they are. Today's slow hip-opening sequence invites you to release stored tension and rest in the truth of your wholeness. We'll move with patience, letting the breath guide the body into deeper ease.

Dragon Pose – Right Side

From an all fours position, step your right foot to the outside of your right hand. Your right foot should be below the knee, and your left toes untucked. Keep your chest lifted and shoulders soft as you sink your hips toward the earth in *Dragon Pose*. Breathe into the stretch you feel in your left hip flexor for one minute, allowing your body to soften and gravity to do the work.

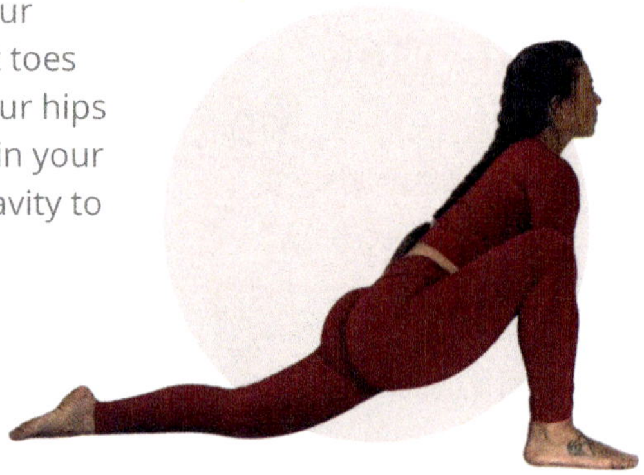

Dragon Pose

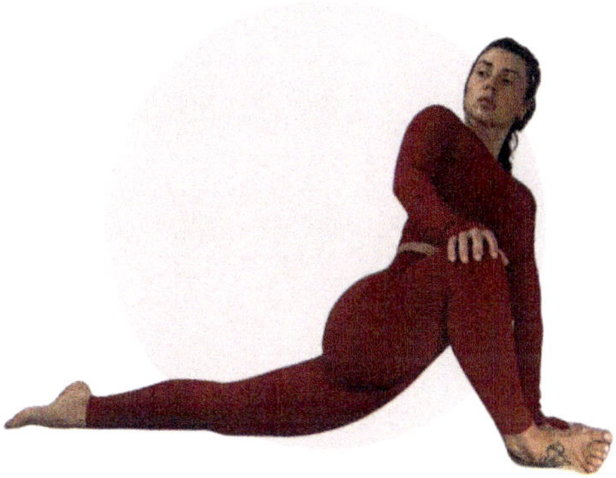

Twisted Dragon

Option to deepen your stretch by taking *Twisted Dragon*. Turn your right toes to face slightly outward, place your right hand on your thigh and gently press the knee out to the side to open the hip. Twist your torso to gaze past your right shoulder. Hold for 1 minute, keeping the breath steady and spacious.

Dragon Pose – Left Side

Step back into *Table Top Pose* before switching sides. Move with care, holding each variation for the same amount of time, and notice any differences between your hips.

Closing

After both sides, come to a comfortable seat. Close your eyes, sensing the openness in your hips, the length in your spine, and the quiet strength within. Silently repeat: *I am already enough*. Carry this truth with you as you step into your day.

Day 9

Theme of the Week: Ground
Quote of the Week: "Root deeply, rise freely."

Theme of the Day: Anchor in Stillness
Quote of the Day: "Your breath is your anchor."

Nadi Shodhana – Alternate Nostril Breathing

Some days, the mind feels like a restless ocean—waves of thought rising and falling without pause. Today's practice offers a way to steady those waters. *Nadi Shodhana* (Alternate Nostril Breathing); is a simple yet powerful pranayama technique that balances the nervous system, harmonizes the left and right hemispheres of the brain, and brings a deep sense of calm. Your breath becomes the anchor that keeps you steady, no matter what currents you encounter.

Finding Your Seat

Begin in a comfortable seated position, cross-legged on the floor, kneeling, or on a chair. Lengthen your spine and allow your shoulders to drop away from your ears. Rest your left hand on your thigh. With your right hand, fold the index and middle fingers toward your palm, keeping the thumb, ring, and pinky finger extended.

The Breathwork Practice

Take a cleansing breath to begin, deep inhale through the nose, and long exhale out of the mouth. Close your right nostril with your thumb and inhale slowly through the left. At the top of the inhale, close the left nostril with your ring finger, release the right nostril, and exhale fully. Inhale through the right nostril, close it with

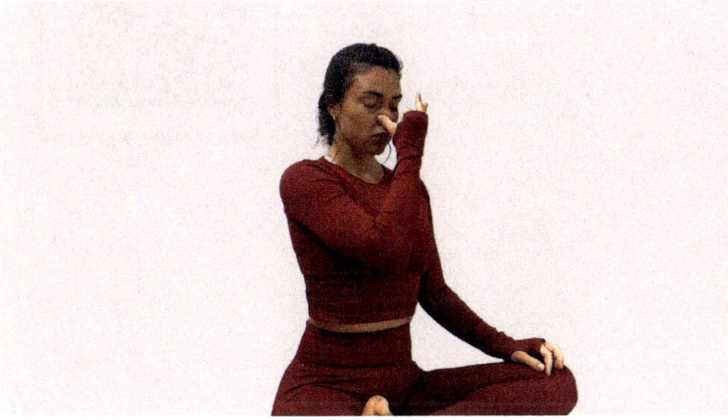

Nadhi Shodhana Thumb Plug

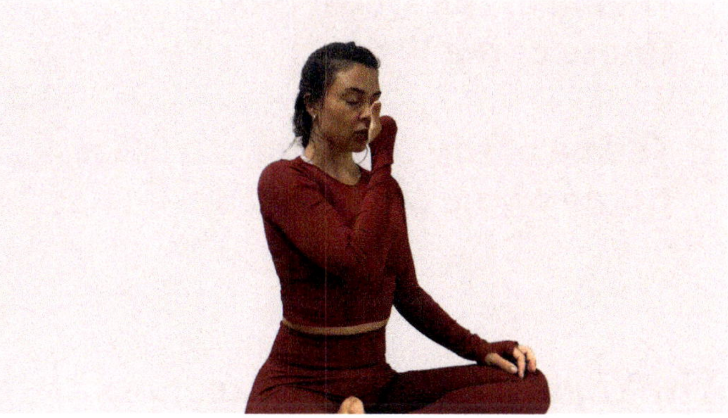

Nadhi Shodhana Ring Finger Plug

your thumb, and exhale through the left. This completes one round.

Continue for 6–8 slow, mindful rounds. Let the breath be smooth and even, your attention resting on the steady flow of air and the subtle softening of the mind.

Closing

When you finish, release your hand, take a cleansing breath, in through the nose; and out through the mouth and then return to natural breathing. Sit for a few quiet moments, sensing the ease and spaciousness within. Let your breath remind you: peace is not something to chase, it is something you return to.

Day 10

Theme of the Week: Ground
Quote of the Week: "Root deeply, rise freely."

Theme of the Day: Root into Stillness
Quote of the Day: "Presence is the practice."

Yin Yoga for Quiet Awareness

In our busy lives, stillness can feel unfamiliar—or even uncomfortable. Yet it is in slowing down that we re-connect most deeply with ourselves. Today's yin practice is a gentle invitation to pause, soften into the spaces we usually rush past, and notice what is present right now. By bringing full awareness to the body, we train ourselves to live more fully in the moment.

Butterfly Pose (*Baddha Konasana*)

Begin seated with the soles of your feet together, knees dropping gently to the sides. Hold your ankles or feet, lengthening the spine on an inhale. Exhale and allow your back to round naturally as you fold forward, keeping the shoulders soft. If it feels supportive, place a cushion or block beneath your forehead.

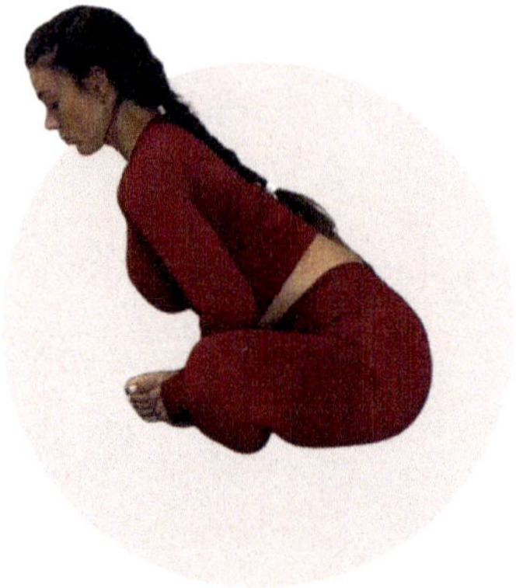

Butterfly Pose

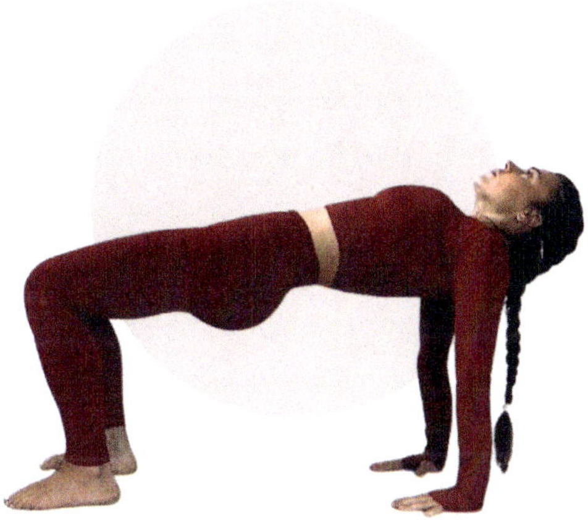

Reverse Tabletop

Close your eyes. Notice the stretch across your inner thighs, the gentle release in your lower back, and the rise and fall of your breath. Stay here for 2 minutes, letting each inhale create space and each exhale invite deeper surrender. If your mind drifts, gently guide it back to the rhythm of your breath.

Counter Stretch – Reverse Tabletop

When ready, sit tall and place your hands behind you, fingers pointing toward your body. Plant your feet hip-width apart. Press through hands and feet to lift your hips, opening the chest toward the sky. Feel your collarbones broaden, shoulders draw back, and front body expand. Breathe deeply for 30 seconds, imagining light filling your chest.

Lower slowly back to a comfortable seat. Take a few quiet breaths, noticing the subtle hum of energy flowing through your body. Let this moment remind you: presence isn't a destination, it is a choice you make, one conscious breath at a time.

Day 11

Theme of the Week: Ground
Quote of the Week: "Root deeply, rise freely."

Theme of the Day: Flow with the Breath
Quote of the Day: "Your breath knows the way."

Hip & Hamstring Slow Flow

Our breath is a constant companion, guiding us through movement, stillness, and transitions. Today's practice uses the rhythm of your inhale and exhale to gently open the hips, lengthen the hamstrings, and create space through the lower body. By moving slowly and mindfully, you'll discover how your breath leads the way—showing you when to deepen, when to soften, and when to pause.

Mountain Pose

Begin by standing tall at the top of your mat, feet hip-width apart, shoulders relaxed, and arms resting gently by your sides. Take a few mindful breaths, feeling your feet root into the earth. With each inhale, imagine your spine lengthening upward; with each exhale, allow your body to soften.

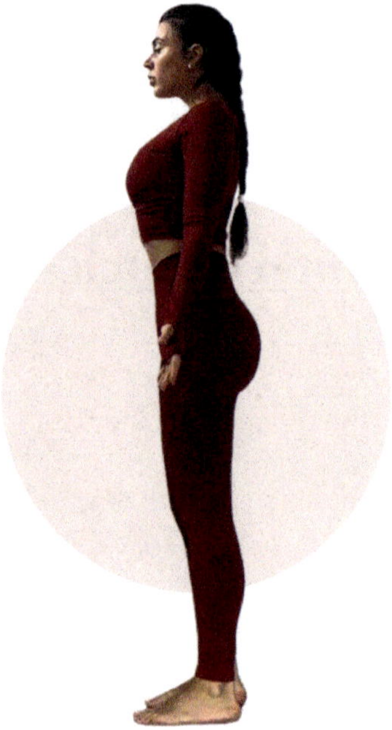

Mountain

Right Side Flow

Plant your hands on the mat and step your left foot to the back of the mat, releasing your left knee to plant in a *Low Lunge*. Inhale, sinking your hips as your chest lifts and spine lengthens.

Exhale, shifting your hips back and straightening your right leg, folding over the front leg into *Half Split*. Move slowly between low lunge and half split for 5 rounds, letting your breath guide the pace and depth of each transition.

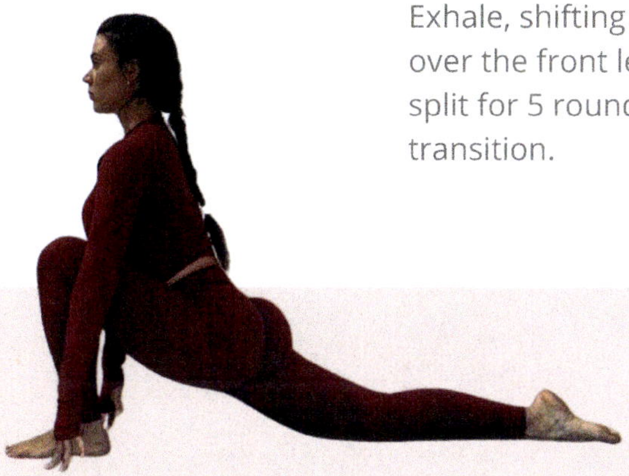

Low Lunge

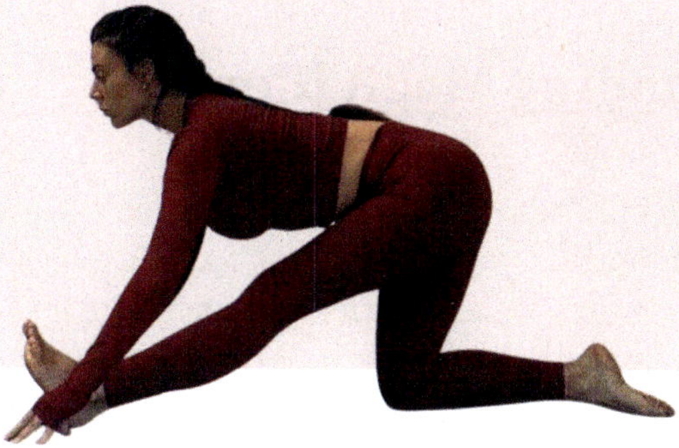

Half Split

Left Side Flow

Return to *Mountain* Pose, pausing for a breath. Repeat the same sequence on the left side, keeping your attention on the breath as it guides each movement—inhale to expand, exhale to soften.

Closing

Return to *Mountain Pose* once more. Close your eyes, noticing the lightness in your legs, the openness in your hips, and the steady rhythm of your breath. Carry this awareness off the mat, trusting that in each moment, your breath truly knows the way.

Day 12

Theme of the Week: Ground
Quote of the Week: "Root deeply, rise freely."

Theme of the Day: Deep Roots, Steady Heart
Quote of the Day: "Let the earth hold you."

Grounding Meditation

Sometimes life moves so quickly that we feel unsteady, like a leaf carried by the wind. Today's practice invites you to reconnect with the steady support beneath your feet and within your body. Through a simple grounding meditation, visualize yourself as a tree, rooting deeply into the earth, and allowing yourself to feel held, supported, and present.

Finding Your Seat

Sit comfortably on the floor, on a cushion, or in a chair with your feet flat on the ground. Rest your hands lightly on your thighs, relax your shoulders, and lengthen your spine. Close your eyes and take a few slow, deep breaths. With each inhale, invite openness and calm. With each exhale, release tension from your body.

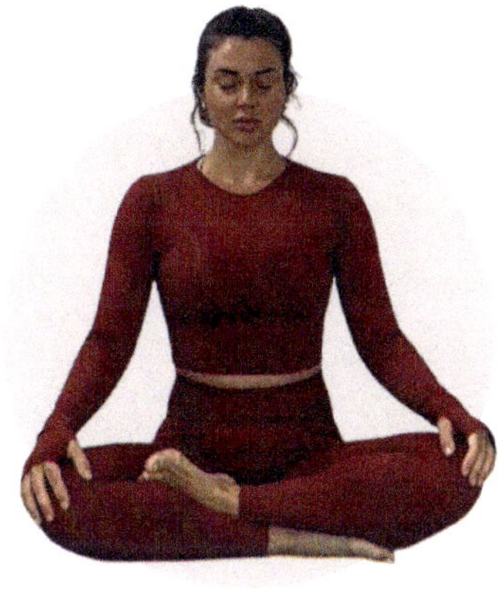

Comfortable Seat Hand to Knees

Tree Visualization

Imagine roots extending from the base of your spine, traveling deep into the earth. With every inhale, draw energy up the body, feeling the strength and stability rising from the ground. With each exhale, send any stress, worry, or tension down through your roots, releasing it safely into the earth.

Visualize your trunk growing tall and steady, branches reaching upward and outward. Your body is both supported and expansive; rooted yet free. Stay here for several minutes, moving only with the gentle rhythm of your breath.

Closing

Slowly bring awareness back to your physical body, noticing the sensations in your feet, legs, and spine. Open your eyes softly, keeping the feeling of grounding with you. Let this meditation remind you that, no matter what unfolds today, the earth is always beneath you, ready to hold and support you. Take one final, deep breath and repeat silently: *I am rooted. I am supported. I am present.*

Day 13

Theme of the Week: Ground
Quote of the Week: "Root deeply, rise freely."

Theme of the Day: Strength in Stillness
Quote of the Day: "Stillness speaks louder than noise."

Squat in Stillness

In our fast-paced lives, moments of stillness can feel rare or even uncomfortable. Today's practice invites you to slow down and cultivate presence through *Malasana* (*Yogi Squat*). This posture opens the hips, strengthens the lower body, and creates a space for reflection and inner quiet. By holding the pose mindfully, we discover that profound growth often comes not from action, but from simply being.

Malasana

Begin standing with feet hip-width apart, toes pointing slightly outward. Slowly bend the knees and lower your hips toward the ground into *Malasana*, keeping your heels planted. If necessary, place either blocks or a rolled towel under the heels for extra support. Press your palms together at your heart center, elbows gently pressing against your inner thighs to encourage hip opening. Lengthen your spine, lift your chest,

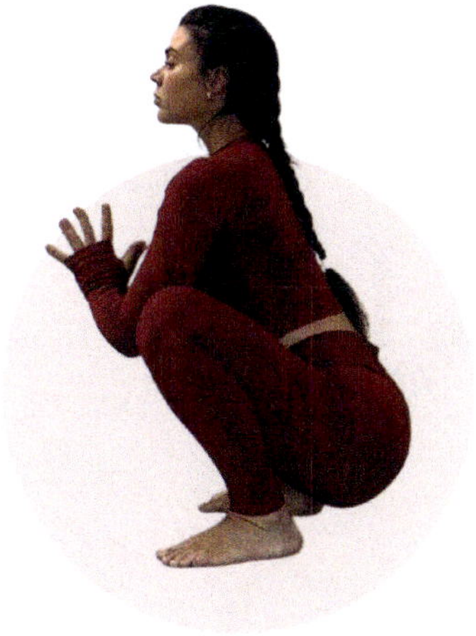

Malasana

and soften your shoulders.

Holding the Pose

Close your eyes and breathe slowly and evenly. Notice the sensations in your hips, ankles, and lower back. With each inhale, draw energy upward through your body. With each exhale, release tension, allowing yourself to melt deeper into the posture without forcing. Stay here for 2 minutes, maintaining steady breath and mindful attention. If your mind wanders, gently return your focus to the grounding, supported presence in your body.

Closing

Slowly rise from the squat into a comfortable standing position. Notice how your body feels—more open, balanced, and aware. Let the stillness cultivated here extend beyond your practice, reminding you that silence and presence often hold more power than constant motion or noise. Carry this awareness into the day, letting your breath and rooted presence guide you. Repeat silently: *I am still. I am grounded. I am present.*

Week 3:

OPEN

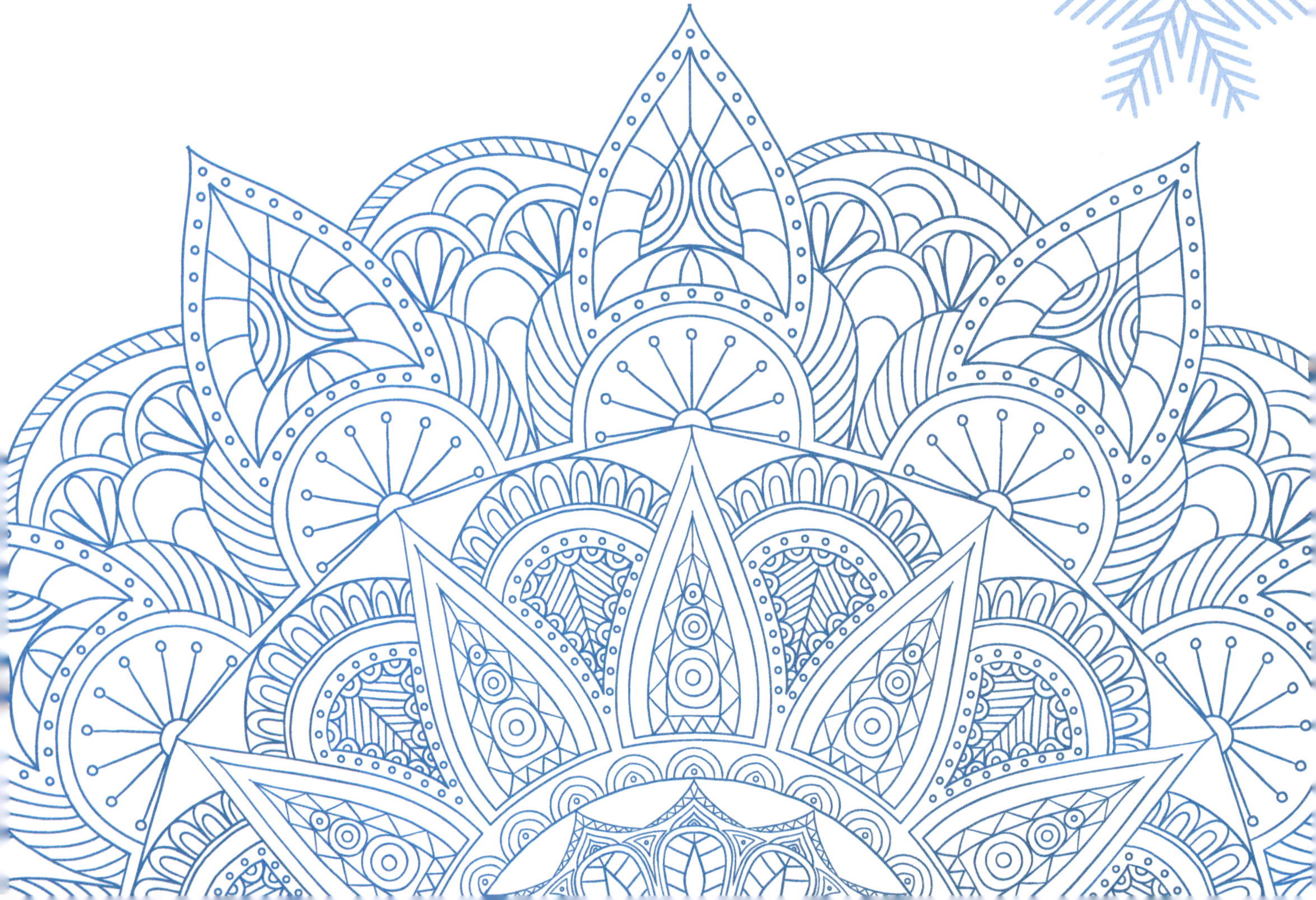

Quote of the Week:

"What is open can receive."

By the time you arrive in Week 3, you've awakened your awareness and rooted yourself in grounding practices. Now the invitation is to **open**. The holidays are a time of giving and receiving, but often we forget that to truly receive, whether it's joy, love, rest, or even breath, we must first soften and open.

Openness is not about pushing your body into deep stretches or forcing your heart to expand. It's about cultivating a gentle willingness: to let go of what weighs you down, to soften protective layers, and to allow yourself to experience the fullness of life as it is in this moment.

This week's practices days 14-20, are designed to invite openness into both the body and the heart. Through gentle backbends, expansive breathing, and meditative awareness, you'll explore what it means to create space physically, mentally, and emotionally. Yin-style holds will help melt away layers of tension across the chest and hips, while guided breathwork and meditation will encourage you to release resistance and welcome in ease.

As you open, you may notice how much more you can receive. A deeper breath. A sense of gratitude. A quiet moment of peace in the midst of a busy day. The practice of opening is not about perfection or achievement—it's about allowing yourself to be receptive, to welcome in lightness, and to create room for joy to settle in.

This week, let openness be your guide. Soften your body, quiet your mind, and open your heart. When you are open, you can receive the gifts of this season, not just in what's given to you, but in the moments you allow yourself to truly feel.

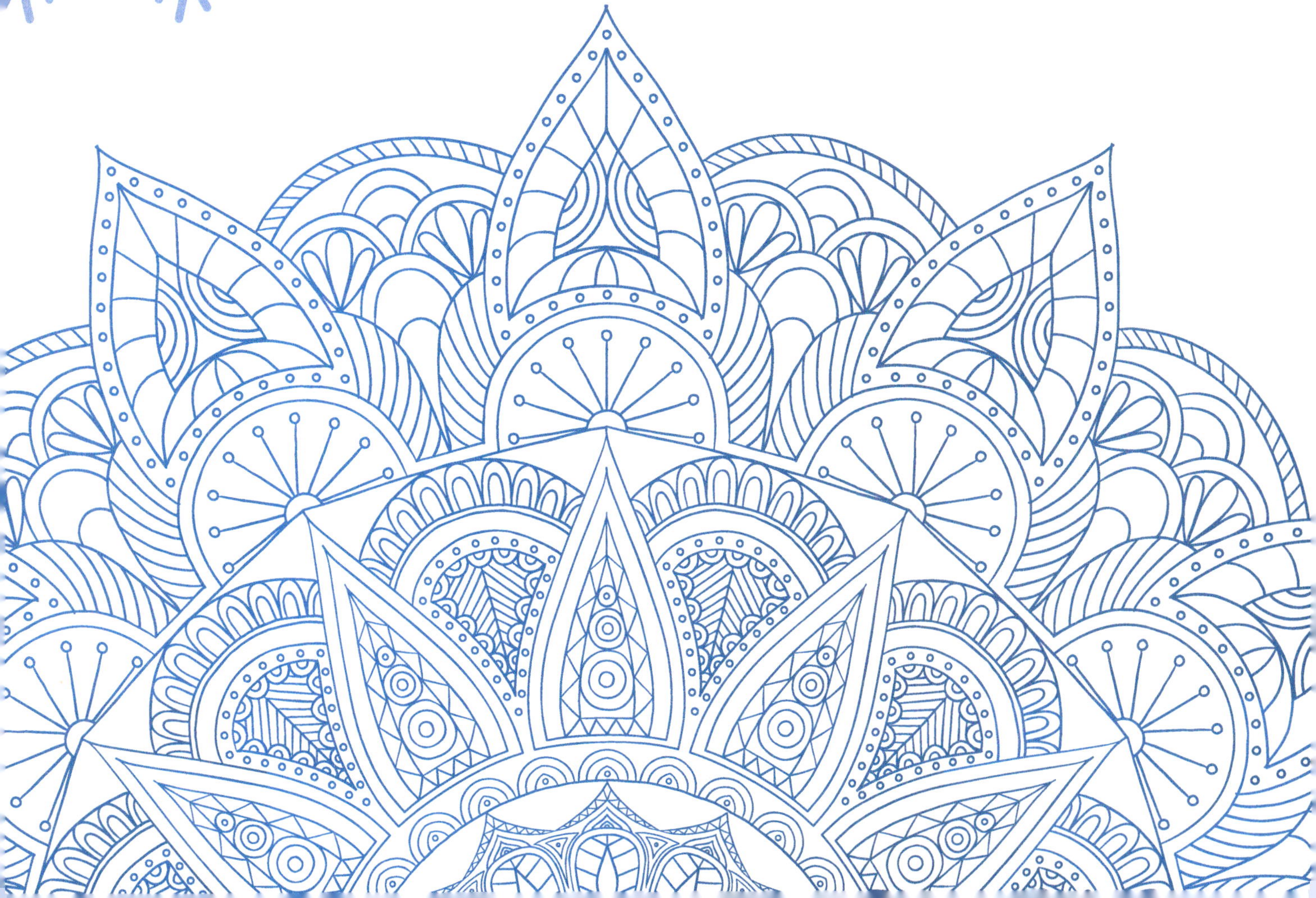

Day 14

Theme of the Week: Open
Quote of the Week: "What is open can receive."

Theme of the Day: Open the Heart
Quote of the Day: "Let your open heart be your guide."

Backbend Boost

Today's practice invites gentle expansion through the spine and heart. Backbends are a beautiful way to release tension stored in the chest and shoulders, encourage energy flow through the front body, and cultivate a sense of openness and gratitude. When held mindfully, each posture becomes a meditative prayer, honoring the body and breath as sacred tools for presence.

Sphinx Pose

Begin lying on your belly with legs extended behind you, and the tops of your feet pressing gently into the mat. Place your forearms on the floor, elbows under your shoulders, palms flat. Press into your forearms as you lift your chest, drawing the shoulder blades down and back. Keep your neck long and gaze forward or slightly down.

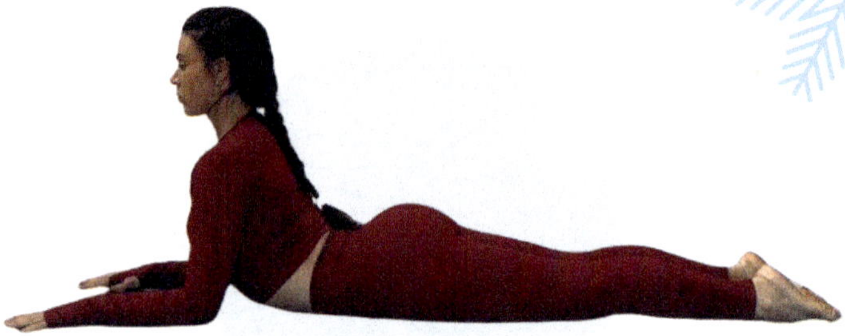

Sphinx Pose

Breathe slowly and evenly as you hold *Sphinx Pose* for 2 minutes, feeling a gentle arch in the spine and openness in the chest. Let each inhale expand your heart space, and each exhale soften your lower back.

Optional Seal Pose

If comfortable, turn your fingers slightly outward and press your palms into the mat straightening your arms to lift higher into *Seal Pose*. Allow the chest to shine forward and upward, deepening the stretch. Hold for an additional minute, breathing fully and evenly. Notice any areas of release or expansion, letting the breath guide your depth rather than forcing the body.

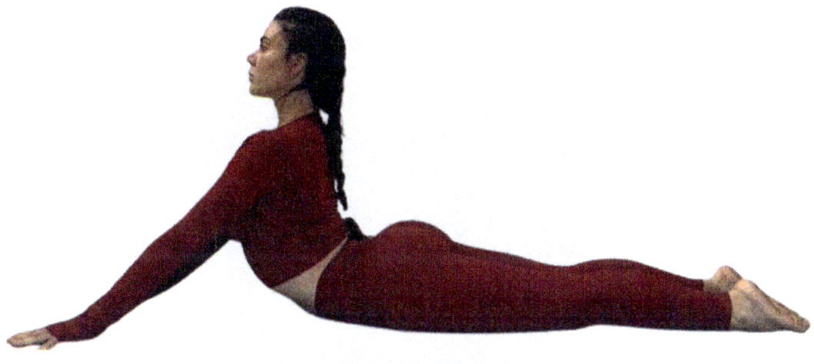

Seal Pose

Child's Pose

Slowly lower back down. Spread the knees apart and press your hips back to *Child's Pose*, releasing the lower back. Reflect on the idea that your yoga practice is more than movement; it is an offering, a prayer, and a reminder of your connection to yourself and the present moment.

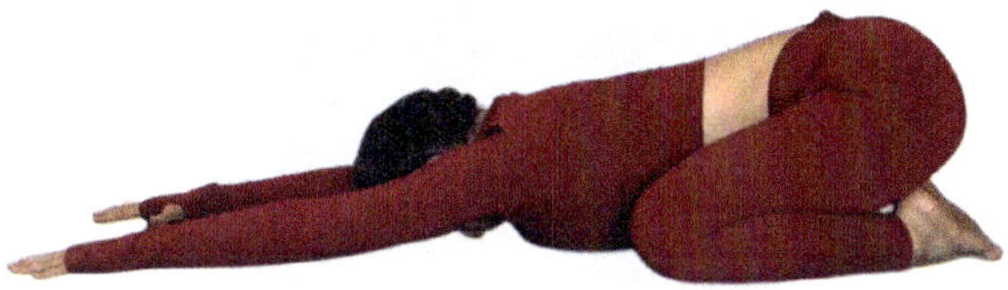

Child's Pose

Carry this openness into your day. Let every breath, and mindful pause remind you: *Let your open heart be your guide.*

Day 15

Theme of the Week: Open
Quote of the Week: "What is open can receive."

Theme of the Day: Surrender and Receive
Quote of the Day: "Let go to receive."

Supported Heart-Opening

Sometimes the deepest gifts come not from effort, but from release. Today's practice invites you to surrender into support, allowing the body and mind to soften fully. *Supported Fish Pose* gently opens the chest, shoulders, and spine while creating space for reflection, self-compassion, and receptivity. By holding this posture mindfully, we practice letting go—releasing tension, control, and rigidity—so that nourishment, clarity, and peace may naturally flow in.

Supported Fish Pose

Find a quiet space and place a bolster, or a rolled blanket, on your mat. Sit in front of the support, then slowly lie back so that your upper back and shoulders rest on it. Let your head be supported by a block or a folded blanket if needed. Legs can extend long on the floor or bend at the knees with feet flat; whichever feels most comfortable. Rest your arms gently outward, palms facing upward, inviting surrender.

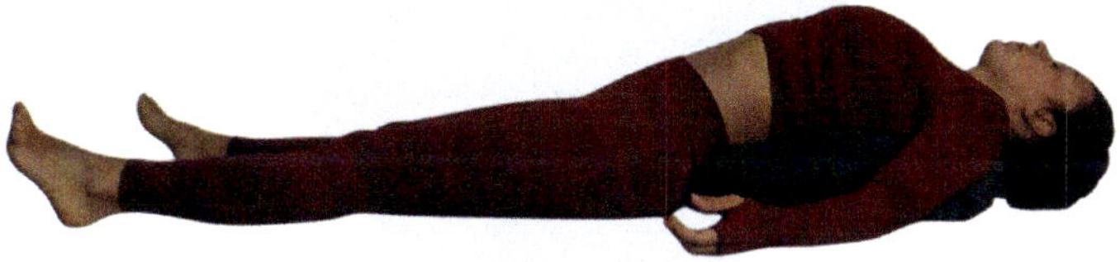

Supported Fish Pose

Holding the Pose

Close your eyes and take deep, steady breaths. With each inhale, feel the chest expand. With each exhale, soften further into the support beneath you. Stay here for 2 minutes, allowing the body to release tension and the mind to settle into stillness. Notice the sensations in the chest, shoulders, and spine, and welcome any emotions or thoughts that arise without judgment.

Closing

When ready, come up to a comfortable seat. Take a moment to honor yourself for this practice, for your surrender, and for the presence you brought to this moment. Carry today's intention with you: letting go creates the space to receive life's gifts fully and openly.

Repeat silently: *I let go. I receive. I am open.*

Day 16

Theme of the Week: Open
Quote of the Week: "What is open can receive."

Theme of the Day: Open Your Heart
Quote of the Day: "Let love lead the way."

Open Heart Flow

Today's practice invites gentle expansion through the chest, shoulders, and spine, creating space for openness and compassion. The heart is not only a physical center but also a doorway to connection—with yourself, others, and the world around you. By moving mindfully with your breath, this flow reminds you that love begins within and naturally radiates outward.

Mountain Pose

Begin standing tall in *Mountain Pose*. Feet grounded, shoulders relaxed, and spine long. Close your eyes briefly, and notice the natural rhythm of your breath. Feel the stability of your feet as they root into the earth, supporting the expansion of your chest and heart.

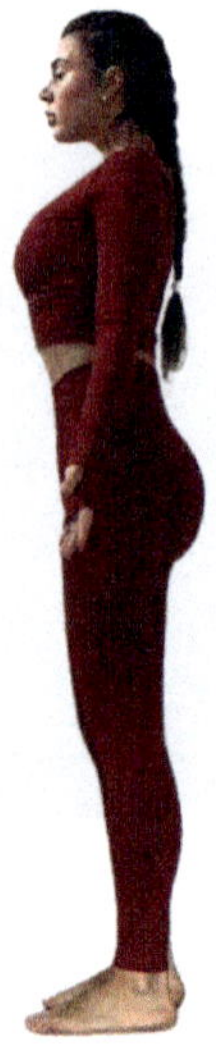

Mountain

Standing Cat-Cow Variation with Cactus Arms

Inhale, lifting your chest and arching the spine while drawing the arms into cactus shape (elbows bent at 90 degrees, palms facing forward), opening the chest. Exhale, round your spine and gently draw your

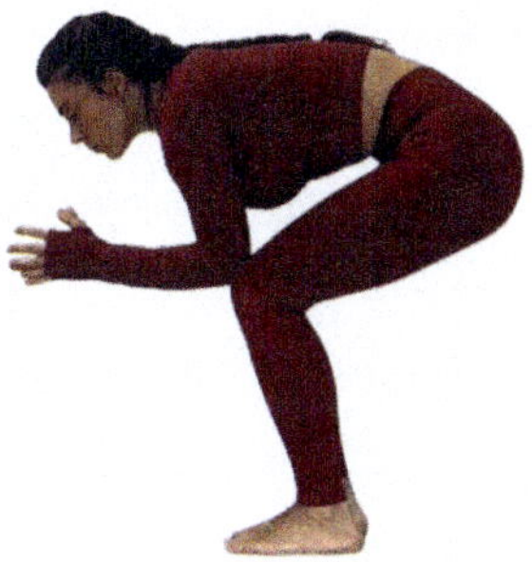

Cactus Cat

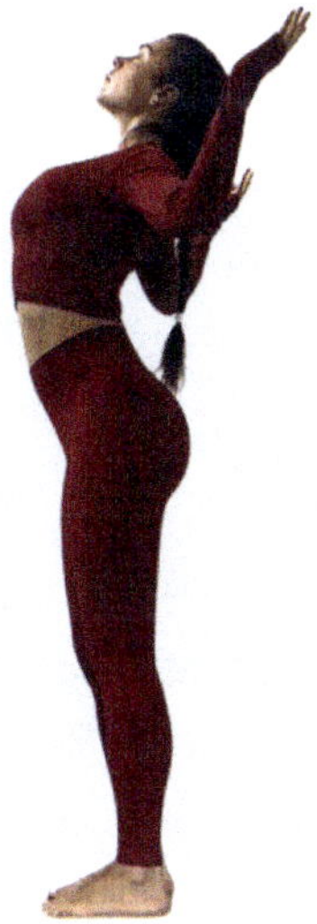

Cactus Cow

forearms together as you slowly bend your knees. Repeat slowly for 5 mindful rounds, synchronizing breath with motion.

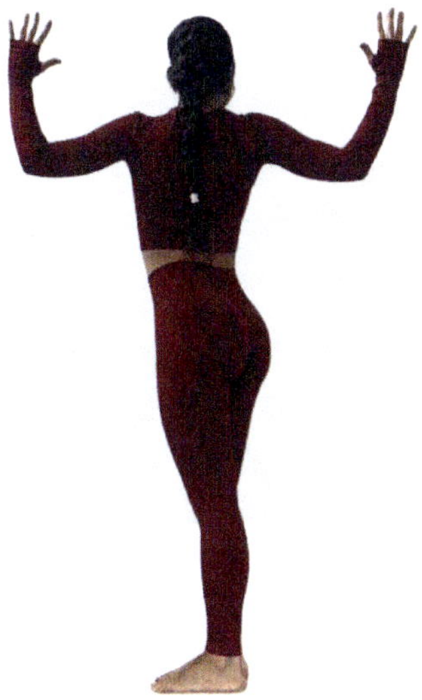

Cactus Twsts

Add Twists

Inhale to open into your cactus arms but this time, twisting to the right, gazing past the right shoulder. Exhale coming back through to center, rounding the spine, forearms together as you bend at the knees curling into a ball. Inhale cactus twist left, then exhale rounding through to center. Continue to move mindfully with the breath until you complete 3 rounds on each side.

Closing in Mountain Pose

Return to standing in *Mountain Pose*. Take a few breaths, feeling the openness in your chest and the grounding through your feet. Let this feeling of heart expansion guide your intentions and interactions throughout the day. Carry this reminder with you: love begins within, and by nurturing it, you allow it to flow naturally into every part of your life. Repeat silently: *I open my heart. I let love lead the way.*

Day 17

Theme of the Week: Open
Quote of the Week: "What is open can receive."

Theme of the Day: Energize with Breath
Quote of the Day: "I breathe, I expand, I receive."

Three-Part Breath

Sometimes the simplest practices are the most profound. *Dirga Pranayama (Three-Part Breath)*; invites awareness into the full capacity of your lungs by consciously breathing into the belly, ribcage, and chest. This practice clears stagnation, revitalizes your nervous system, and creates space in both body and mind. Through gentle focus, you'll feel grounded and centered, while also expanding your energy outward with clarity and ease.

Finding Your Space

Come to a comfortable seated position, cross-legged on the ground or supported on a block or pillow. If seated in a chair, rest your feet flat on the ground. Lengthen your spine, soften your shoulders, and gently close your eyes. Place one hand on the belly and the other on the heart, drawing your attention inward.

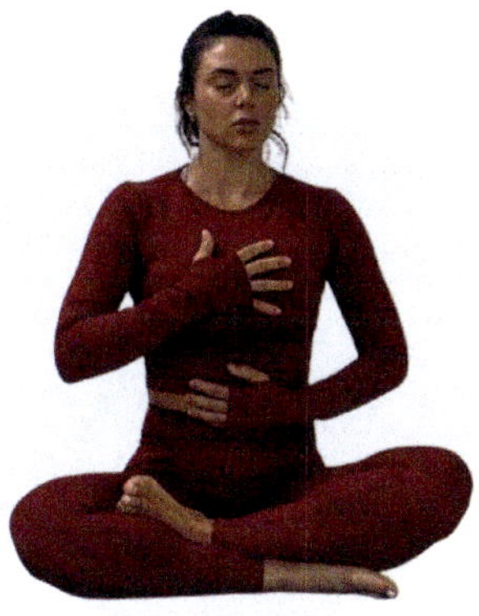

Comfortable Seat Hand to Belly & Heart

The Practice

Inhale slowly through the nose, first filling the belly and feeling it rise under your hand. Continue the inhale into the ribcage, expanding outward. Finally, sip the breath all the way into the chest, lifting gently through the heart space. Pause briefly at the top, then exhale steadily, releasing from the chest, ribs, and belly in reverse order. Continue this slow, mindful pattern for several rounds, letting the rhythm of breath carry you into stillness and vitality.

Focus and Awareness

Notice how each inhale creates expansion and space, while each exhale releases tension and grounds you in the present. Keep the face soft, the shoulders relaxed, and the breath unhurried. Allow the practice to feel nourishing rather than effortful, finding a natural balance between expansion and release.

Closing

Rest your hands gently in your lap or by your sides. Sit quietly and observe the subtle shift in your energy — a calm clarity, a sense of openness in the heart and mind. Carry this awareness into the rest of your day, remembering that breath is your anchor and your source of renewal. Repeat silently: *I breathe. I expand. I receive.*

Day 18

Theme of the Week: Open
Quote of the Week: "What is open can receive."

Theme of the Day: Surrender to Peace
Quote of the Day: "The art of surrender is the path to peace."

Heart Melt

Today's practice invites gentle release through the chest, shoulders, and spine, cultivating a deep sense of surrender and calm. *Uttana Shishosana (Puppy Pose)*; opens the heart space while allowing the body and mind to soften. True peace arises not from effort, but from surrender. By holding this posture mindfully, we create room for rest, clarity, and emotional release.

Puppy Pose

Begin on all fours in a Table Top position, knees under hips and hands under shoulders. Slowly walk your hands forward, lowering your chest toward the mat while keeping hips stacked above your knees. Rest your forehead or chin on the mat, letting your arms extend fully or slightly bent, whichever feels most comfortable. Close your eyes and take a few deep, grounding breaths.

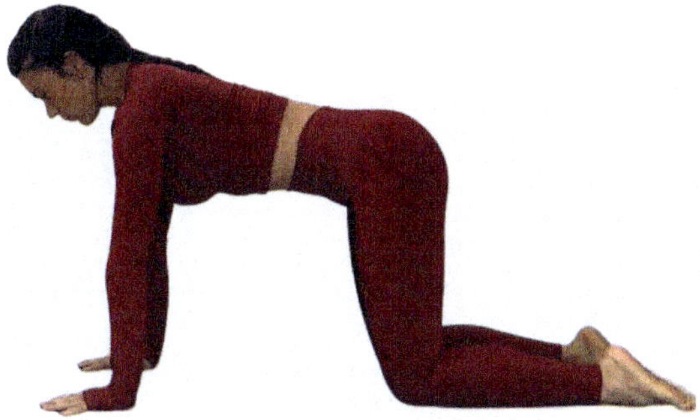

Table Top

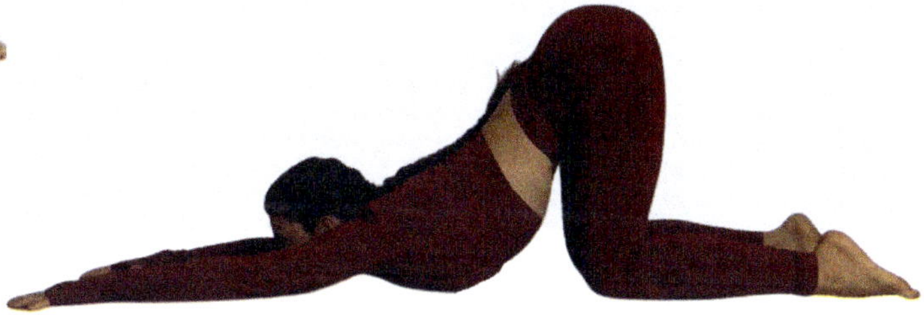

Puppy Pose

Holding the Pose

Stay here for 2 full minutes, letting the breath guide the depth of the stretch. With each inhale, imagine opening the heart, expanding the chest, and drawing energy upward. With each exhale, allow tension, resistance, or worry to melt away into the mat. Notice any tightness or discomfort and greet it with acceptance, remembering that surrender is not weakness, it is a conscious release.

Closing

When ready, gently walk your hands back toward your body, and come to a comfortable seated position. Observe the sensations in your chest, shoulders, and spine, and notice the subtle shifts in your mental and emotional state. Let the stillness and openness cultivated here carry with you beyond the mat. Reflect silently: *I surrender. I release. I am at peace.*

Let today's practice serve as a reminder that softening and opening creates space for calm, clarity, and connection—to yourself, the present moment, and life itself.

Day 19

Theme of the Week: Open
Quote of the Week: "What is open can receive."

Theme of the Day: Power in Vulnerability
Quote of the Day: "Vulnerability is your power."

Mantra Meditation

Today's practice invites you to explore the strength in vulnerability. By combining breath with mantra, we can anchor the mind, open the heart, and cultivate the courage to be fully present. Repeating a simple phrase with conscious breathing allows tension to release, mental chatter to quiet, and the power of authentic presence to emerge.

Finding Your Seat

Sit comfortably on the floor, on a cushion, or in a chair with your feet grounded. Lengthen your spine and relax your shoulders, resting your hands gently on your thighs or knees, palms facing upward. Close your eyes and take a few deep, slow breaths, noticing the natural rhythm of your inhale and exhale. Allow your body to soften and your mind to settle.

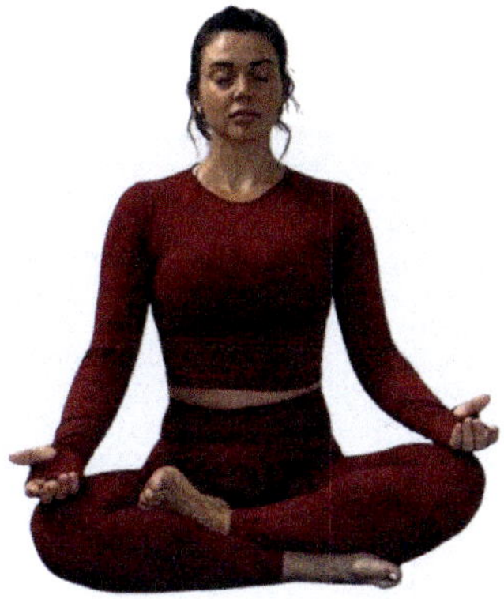

Comfortable Seat Palms Face Upward

The Mantra Practice

On your next inhale, silently say, "I am." On your exhale, complete the phrase with, "open." Let the mantra flow naturally with your breath, creating a gentle, steady rhythm. Feel each inhale expand your chest and bring energy to your body. With each exhale, release fear, resistance, or tension, leaving space for openness, compassion, and presence. Continue for several minutes, letting the repetition deepen your connection to yourself.

Reflection and Awareness

Notice that vulnerability is a doorway to authenticity, connection, and inner strength. Observe any subtle shifts in your heart, mind, and body as you repeat "I am open." Feel the courage that arises from allowing yourself to be; fully and without judgment.

Closing

Slowly return to natural breathing, resting your hands in your lap. Take a moment to honor the openness you've cultivated. Carry this intention with you: vulnerability is not weakness; it is your power, a bridge to connection, compassion, and self-acceptance.

Repeat silently: *I am open. I am strong. I am present.*

Day 20

Theme of the Week: Open
Quote of the Week: "What is open can receive."

Theme of the Day: Move like water
Quote of the Day: "I move with ease. I flow with grace. I am present."

Gentle Flow

Today's practice invites you to move with the body's natural rhythm, cultivating flexibility, fluidity, and ease. Gentle transitions between *Child's Pose* and *Cobra Pose* encourage the spine to awaken, the chest to open, and the nervous system to find calm. By flowing mindfully with your breath, you release tension and reconnect with the effortless movement already present within you.

Starting in Child's Pose

Begin in *Child's Pose*, knees spread wide, big toes touching, walking the hands forward, as the hips sit back towards the heels, forehead grounding on the mat. Take a few deep breaths here, noticing the weight of your body sinking into the mat and allowing your mind to soften.

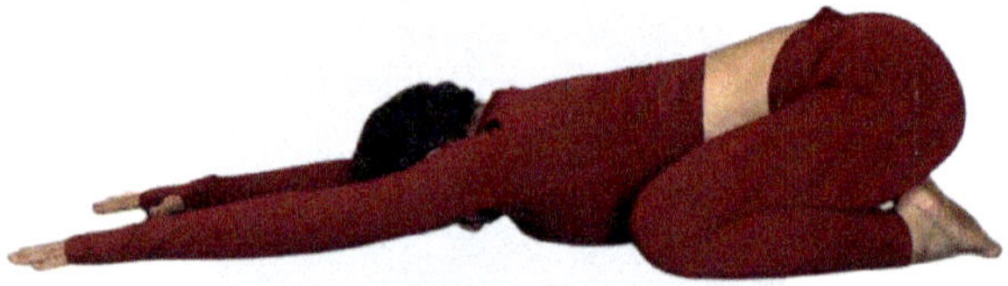

Child's Pose

Transition to Cobra

On an inhale, gently draw your heart forwards and up as your hips melt towards the mat, coming into *Cobra Pose*. Drawing the shoulder blades down your back, feel the gentle arch in your spine and the expansion in your chest. Exhale to lower back down into *Child's Pose*, allowing the spine to lengthen and soften.

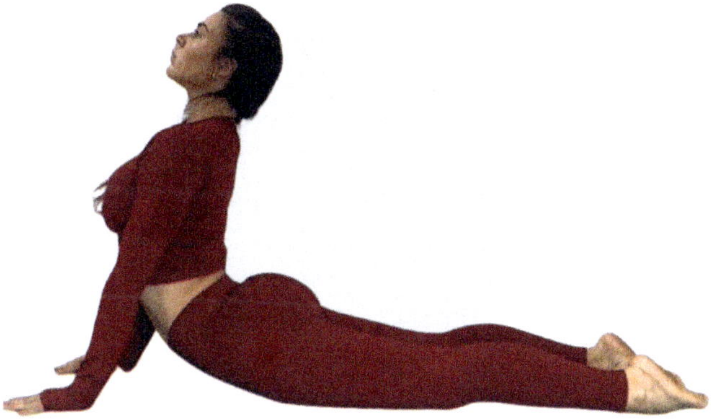

Cobra Pose

Flowing with Breath

Continue this movement for 10 rounds, syncing each transition with deep, intentional breathing. Inhale as you lift into *Cobra Pose*, exhale as you sit back into *Child's Pose*. Focus on the sensations in your spine, chest, and shoulders, noticing how each movement creates more space and fluidity. Release any need to force the stretch or achieve a particular shape; the flow is its own guide.

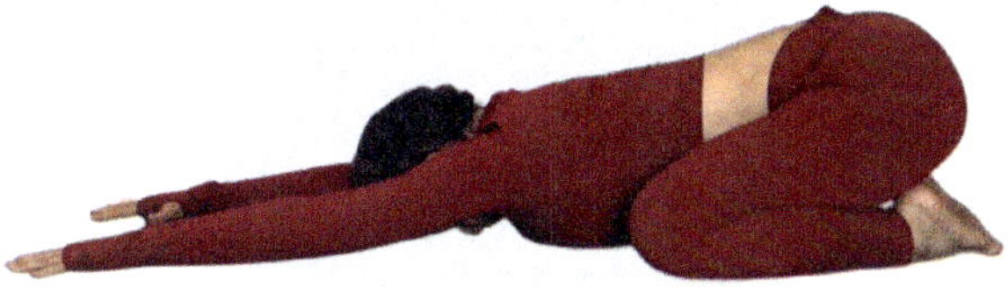

Child's Pose

Closing

After completing the flow, pause in *Child's Pose*. Take a few quiet breaths, reflecting on the ease, fluidity, and openness cultivated in your body. Let this awareness extend beyond your mat: just like water, life flows best without resistance.

Repeat silently: *I move with ease. I flow with grace. I am present.*

Week 4:

RESTORE

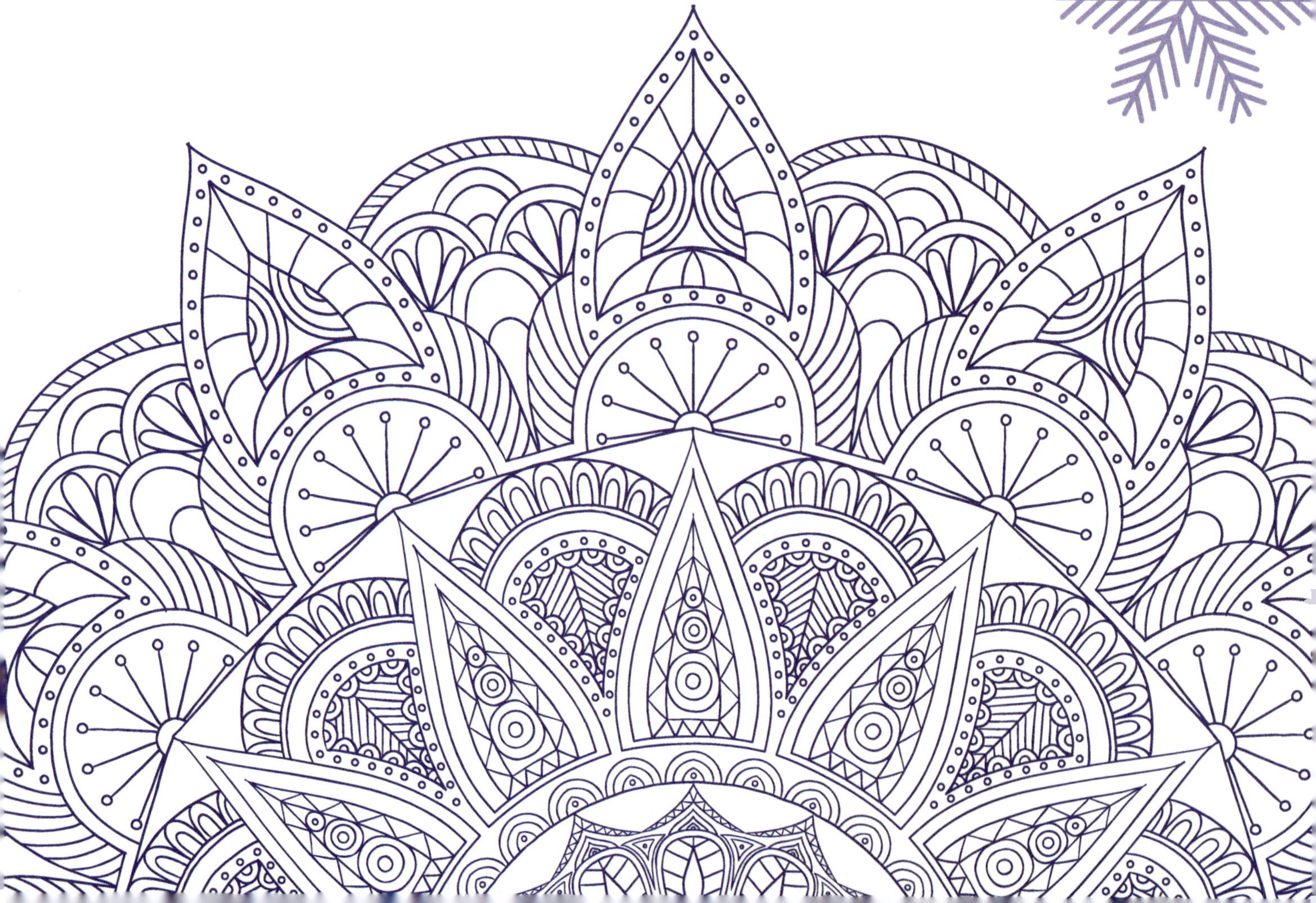

Quote of the Week:

"In stillness,
we find
strength."

As the final days of your Yoga Advent Calendar arrive, the focus turns to **restoration**. The holidays can be joyful, but they are also demanding—on our energy, our schedules, and our emotions. By now, you may feel the pull of the season more deeply. This is why the last step of our journey is to restore: to rest deeply, to replenish your energy, and to allow your body and mind the gift of true recovery.

Restoration is not a luxury; it is essential. Just as the earth rests in winter to prepare for spring, we too must honor the cycles of effort and ease. Without rest, we burn out. With rest, we return to balance, clarity, and vitality.

This week's practices, days 21- 25, will invite you into stillness and softness. You'll explore gentle yin-style postures, calming breathwork, and meditations that soothe the nervous system. Each practice will remind you that rest is not about doing nothing, but about creating the conditions for renewal. In resting, you are nourishing your energy so that you can meet life and the new year ahead with openness and strength.

As you close this journey, notice how far you've come: awakening your awareness, grounding your presence, opening your heart, and now restoring your spirit. This is the natural arc of yoga, and it mirrors the rhythm of life itself.

Let Week 4 be your reminder that rest is not a pause from living, it is living. It is the place where healing happens, where strength is rebuilt, and where the light within you can shine again.

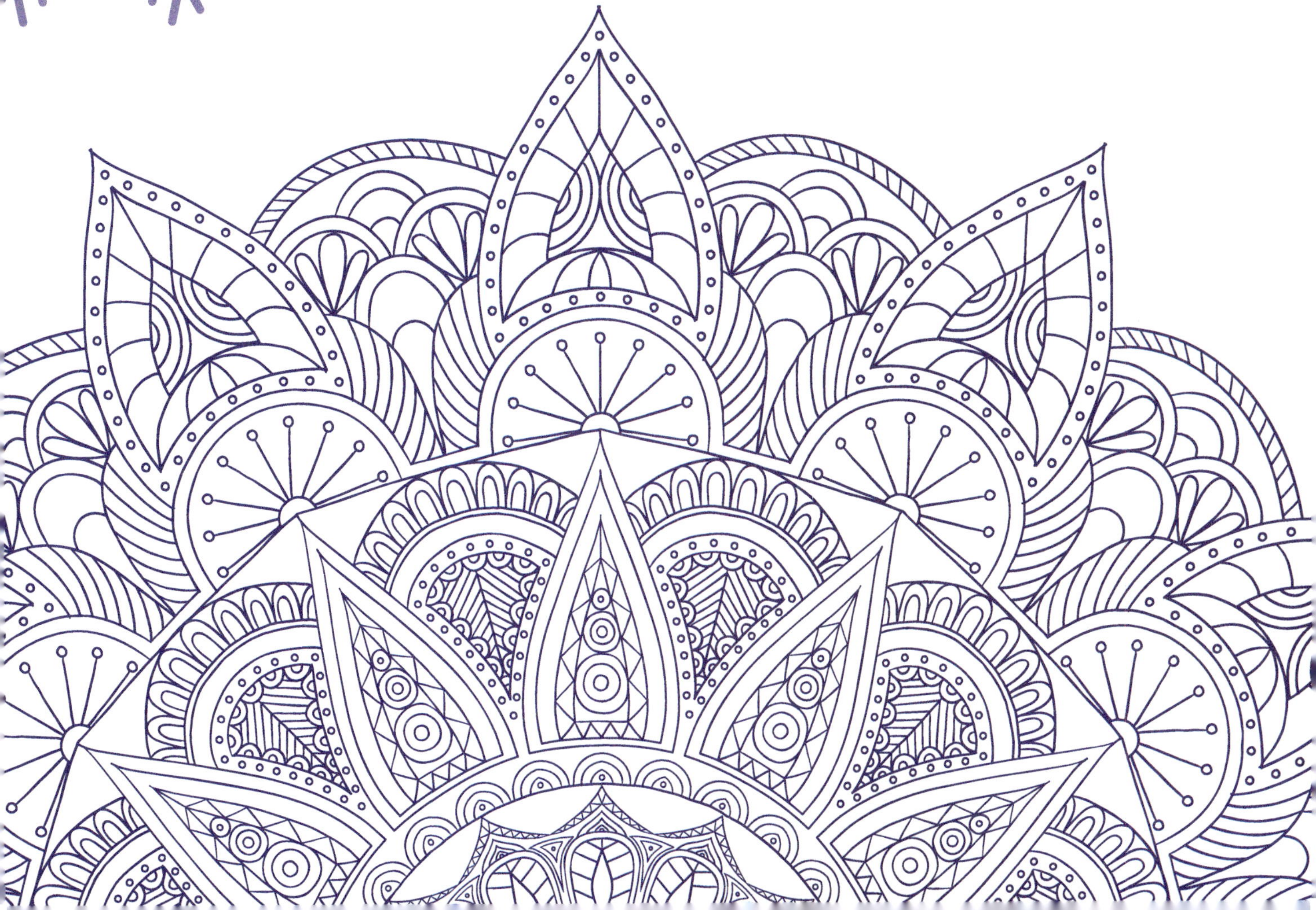

Day 21

Theme of the Week: Restore
Quote of the Week: "Rest to rise."

Theme of the Day: Reconnect with your essence
Quote of the Day: "Come back to yourself."

Simple Inversion for Restoration

Today's practice invites gentle inversion, encouraging the body and mind to rest, restore, and reconnect. *Viparita Karani*; (*Legs Up the Wall*) is a soothing posture that promotes circulation, eases tension in the lower body, and creates a sense of calm and grounding. By turning inward and allowing gravity to support you, this simple inversion becomes a powerful tool to come back to yourself, even amidst life's busyness.

Legs Up the Wall

Find a quiet wall space and place a blanket or cushion underneath your hips for added support if desired. Sit sideways with one hip close to the wall, then gently lie back and swing your legs up to rest vertically against the wall. Allow your arms to rest by your sides, palms open, shoulders soft, and spine long. Close your eyes and take a few deep, grounding breaths, feeling the connection of your back and hips to the floor.

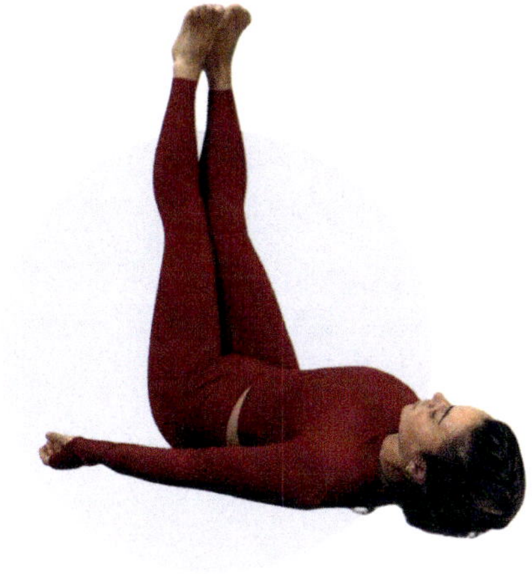

Legs Up the Wall

Restorative Holding

Stay in this position for several minutes, allowing your body to release tension naturally. Notice how your legs feel as they rest, how your spine lengthens, and how your heart begins to feel light and open. With each inhale, imagine drawing fresh energy upward; with each exhale, let go of fatigue, stress, or worry. Let the earth fully support you, offering a reminder that surrender and stillness are not signs of weakness, but paths to restoration.

Closing

When you are ready, gently bend your knees and roll to one side, pausing for a moment before coming up to a comfortable seated position. Take a few final breaths, noticing the sense of calm, balance, and presence that this simple inversion has created. Carry this awareness with you through your day, returning to it whenever you need to reconnect with yourself.

Repeat silently: *I rest. I restore. I heal..*

Day 22

Theme of the Week: Restore
Quote of the Week: "Rest to rise."

Theme of the Day: Gentle Release
Quote of the Day: "Soften into stillness."

Yin Style Reclined Twist

Today's practice invites you to release tension, open your spine, and cultivate a sense of ease through a gentle Yin-style twist. Reclined twists help relieve tightness in the back, shoulders, and hips, while also creating space for emotional and mental release. By moving slowly and holding the posture mindfully, we allow the body and mind to soften, honoring the wisdom that rest and surrender are vital parts of our practice.

Setting Up the Twist

Begin lying in *Savasana*, legs extended and arms resting at your sides.

Right Side Twist

Hug your right knee into your chest, grabbing your outer knee with your left hand, with your right arm extended and resting on the ground

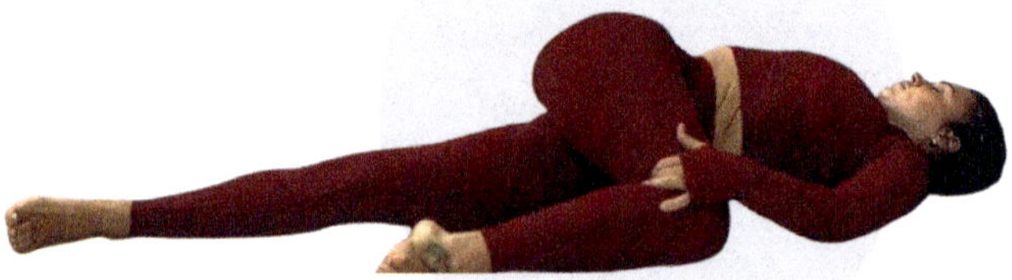

Reclined Twist Right

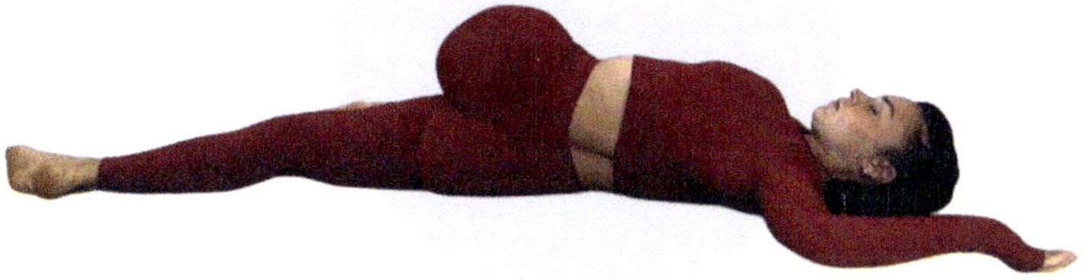

Reclined Twist Left

beside you. From here, draw your knee across your body into a *reclined twist*. Keep both shoulders grounded, letting gravity guide the twist without forcing it. Turn your gaze to the right if it feels comfortable, twisting your spine, opening your outer hip and chest. Close your eyes and breathe deeply, allowing your body to melt into the floor. Stay here for 2 full minutes, noticing any areas of tension and letting each exhale invite release.

Left Side Twist

Return your knee to center and repeat the twist on the left side, maintaining the same mindful awareness and steady breath. Feel the subtle shifts in your spine, hips, and torso as you open into the stretch.

Closing

Make your way back into *Savasana*. Take a few deep, conscious breaths and reflect on the sense of space, softness, and release you have created in your body and mind. When you feel ready, begin to wiggle the fingers and toes re-awakening the body. Roll to your side body in a fetal position, before making your way to a comfortable seat to close off todays practice.

Repeat silently: *I am allowed to soften. I am supported. I am present.*

Let today's practice serve as a reminder that it is not only okay, but essential, to soften, release, and honor the needs of your body and mind.

Day 23

Theme of the Week: Restore
Quote of the Week: "Rest to rise."

Theme of the Day: Calm the Mind and Body
Quote of the Day: "Let your nervous system exhale."

Guided Breath

Today's practice invites you to intentionally slow and lengthen your breath, activating the parasympathetic nervous system and cultivating deep relaxation. By creating a rhythm where the exhale is slightly longer than the inhale, we signal to the body that it is safe to rest, release tension, and return to balance. This simple yet powerful practice calms the mind, steadies emotions, and restores the body.

Finding Your Position

Sit comfortably on the floor, on a cushion, or in a chair with your feet grounded. Rest your hands gently on your thighs or knees. Lengthen your spine, relax your shoulders, and close your eyes. Take a few natural breaths, noticing the rise and fall of your chest and belly.

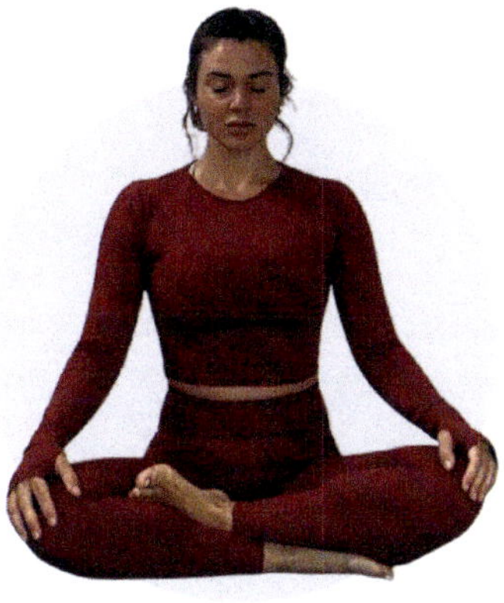

Comfortable Seat Hands to Kness

The Breath Practice- Inhale 4, Exhale 6

Inhale gently through your nose for a count of 4, feeling the belly expand first, then the chest. Pause briefly at the top if it feels natural. Exhale fully and slowly through your nose for a count of 6, releasing any tension, and stress. Continue this pattern for 10 full rounds, letting the breath create a gentle rhythm that soothes and steadies the nervous system.

Awareness and Focus

As you breathe, notice the subtle changes in your body: the softening of your shoulders, the expansion of your chest, the calm settling in your mind. If thoughts arise, observe them; and return your attention to the inhale and exhale. Allow the extended exhale to carry away mental clutter, leaving space for ease and clarity.

Closing

Finish with a cleansing breath. Inhale deeply through the nose; and exhale through the mouth; return to your natural breathing rhythm. Take a moment to acknowledge the calm and balance cultivated through this practice. Let this mindful breathing serve as a reminder that, even amidst a busy day, you can always return to your breath to restore your body and mind.

Repeat silently: *Inhale peace. Exhale stress.*

Day 24

Theme of the Week: Restore
Quote of the Week: "Rest to rise."

Theme of the Day: Embody Peace
Quote of the Day: "Your peace is your power."

Body Scan Guided Meditation

Today's practice invites you to cultivate full-body awareness and deep relaxation through a gentle body scan. By bringing mindful attention to each part of your body, you release tension, reconnect with your physical self, and anchor your awareness in the present moment. This meditation encourages the understanding that peace is not something outside of you; it is found within, and it is a source of strength.

Finding Your Space

Lie down comfortably on your back in *Savasana*, using a mat, blanket, or cushion for support. Let your legs rest naturally, arms by your sides, palms open toward the sky. Close your eyes and take a few slow, grounding breaths, noticing the natural rhythm of your body. Allow yourself to settle fully into the support beneath you.

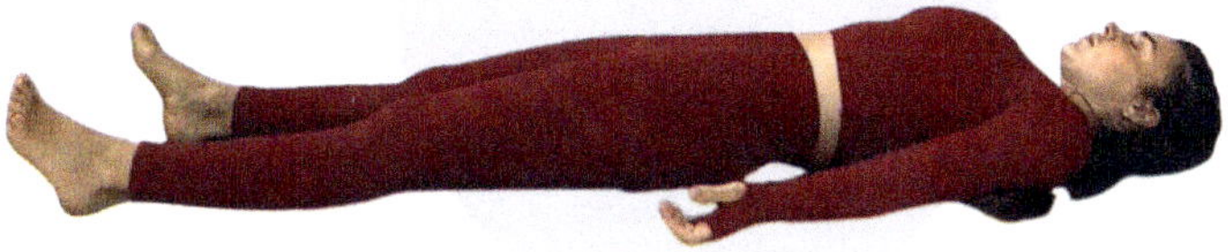

Savasana

Guided Scan

Begin by bringing gentle awareness to the bottoms of your feet, noticing any sensations; or tightness. See if you can allow the feet to soften and relax. Slowly move your focus to your lower legs, knees, upper legs, and hips, observing without judgment. Inhale drawing fresh oxygen into the body, exhale, and feel yourself melt deeper into the mat.

Move attention to your torso, shoulders, and arms. Eventually moving through your neck, face, and head. Feel the connection of your body to the earth, noticing where you carry tension and where you feel spaciousness. Allow your breath to flow naturally as you guide awareness from the bottoms of the feet all the way to the crown of the head, embracing a sense of peace, and presence.

Closing

Once your scan is complete, take a few full breaths, feeling the body fully supported and your mind calm. Slowly wiggle your fingers and toes, stretch lightly if needed, and roll to one side before coming to a comfortable seated position. Reflect on the idea that your inner peace is a source of power, guiding your actions, thoughts, and presence in the world.

Repeat silently: *I am aware. I am relaxed. My peace is my power.*

Let today's practice be a gentle reminder that grounding in your body and mind strengthens you, centers you, and allows your calm presence to shine outward.

Day 25

Theme of the Week: Restore
Quote of the Week: "Rest to rise."

Theme of the Day: Replenish and Restore
Quote of the Day: "Replenish, reconnect, restore."

Rest in Gratitude

Today's practice is a gentle, restorative conclusion to your Advent journey. By combining a deep hip opener with a nurturing *Savasana* focused on gratitude, we create space for reflection, release, and replenishment. This practice encourages connection—to your body, your breath, and the present moment—reminding you that restoration is an essential part of growth and well-being.

Reclined Figure 4 Stretch

Begin lying on your back with knees bent and feet flat on the mat. Cross your right ankle over your left thigh, forming a "4" shape. Flex the right foot to protect the knee and gently draw the left thigh toward your chest, feeling a deep stretch in the

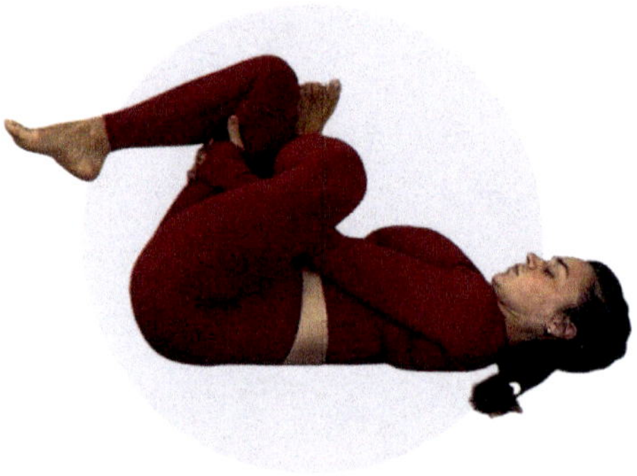

Reclined Figure 4

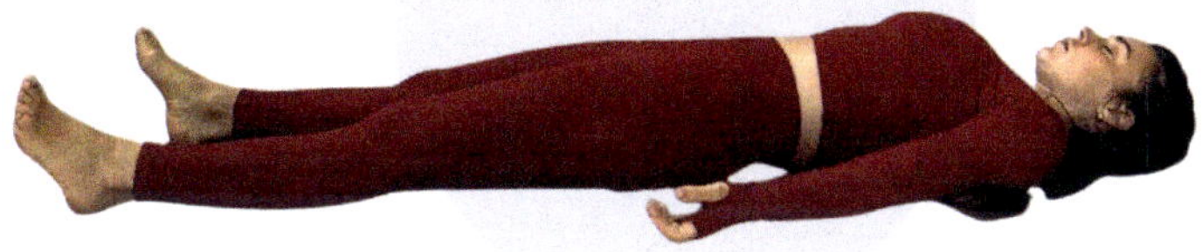

Savasana

right hip. Hold for 1 minute, breathing fully and letting go of tension. Switch sides, crossing the left ankle over the right thigh and drawing the right leg in, maintaining mindful awareness and openness throughout the stretch.

Savasana

After your stretches, release your legs long on the mat and settle into *Savasana*. Let your arms rest comfortably by your sides, palms facing up, and close your eyes. Take a few deep breaths, allowing your body to melt into the ground beneath you. Bring awareness to any, sensations in your body. Feel gratitude for your breath that has carried you through this journey. Reflect on the things you are grateful for, big or small, and let every inhale invite gratitude and positive energy, while each exhale releases anything that you are ready to let go of. Stay in *Savasana* for 2 minutes, allowing your mind to soften and your body to restore.

Closing

When you feel ready, begin to wiggle your fingers and toes, stretch gently, and roll to one side before rising to a comfortable seated position. Take a final moment to place your hands over your heart, honoring yourself for the dedication, presence, and care you have brought to your body and mind during this Advent journey.

Repeat silently: *I replenish. I reconnect. I restore.*

Carry this sense of restoration, gratitude, and openness with you, knowing that the benefits of your practice extend far beyond the mat into your daily life.

We'd love your feedback!

Thank you for joining this Yoga Advent journey!

Your experience matters to us - and we'd love to hear your thoughts.

If you have any **suggestions for improvement**, or if you notice that a **QR code isn't working properly**, please let us know.

You can contact us at: **info@bookshelter-books.com**

Your feedback helps us make each edition even better.

Thank you for your time and your positive energy!

Printed in Dunstable, United Kingdom

73484256R00045